PRESCRIBING OUR FUTURE

PRESCRIBING OUR FUTURE
Ethical Challenges in Genetic Counseling

Dianne M. Bartels, Bonnie S. LeRoy, and
Arthur L. Caplan
EDITORS

ALDINE DE GRUYTER
New York

About the Editors

Dianne M. Bartels is Associate Director, Center for Biomedical Ethics, University of Minnesota. A member of the University of Minnesota's Biomedical Ethics Committee since 1982, she is also a founding member of the Minnesota Network of Institutional Ethics Committees. She is a coauthor of *Beyond Baby M: Ethical Issues in New Reproductive Techniques.*

Bonnie S. LeRoy is a Genetic Counselor, Director of the Graduate Program in Genetic Counseling, and Associate of the Center for Biomedical Ethics, University of Minnesota. Her interests include psychosocial, ethical, and legal issues in genetic counseling. She has published numerous journal articles.

Arthur L. Caplan is Director, Center for Biomedical Ethics, University of Minnesota. A professor of Surgery and Philosophy, he is the author of numerous books and over 300 journal articles. Among his most recent books are *If I Were a Rich Man Could I Buy a Pancreas, and Other Essays on Medical Ethics; When Medicine Went Mad: Bioethics and the Holocaust; Scientific Controversies;* and (is a coauthor) *Beyond Baby M: Ethical Issues in New Reproductive Techniques.*

ALDINE DE GRUYTER
A division of Walter de Gruyter, Inc.
200 Saw Mill River Road
Hawthorne, New York 10532

This publication is printed on acid-free paper ∞

Library of Congress Cataloging-in-Publication Data

Prescribing our future: ethical challenges in genetic counseling/
    edited by Dianne M. Bartels, Bonnie S. LeRoy and Arthur L. Caplan.
        p. cm.
    Includes bibliographical references and index.
    ISBN 0-202-30452-3 (acid-free paper).—ISBN 0-202-30453-1 (pbk.
: acid-free paper)
    1. Genetic counseling—Moral and ethical aspects. I. Bartels,
Dianne M. II. LeRoy, Bonnie. III. Caplan, Arthur L.
RB155.7.P74 1993
174'.2—dc20   OCLC: 2676 2749   92-21469
                                                        CIP

Manufactured in the United States of America

10 9 8 7 6 5 4 3 2 1

Contents

III. Future Directions and Ethical Challenges in Genetic Counseling

IV. Appendix

List of Contributors

Charles L. Bosk

Department of Sociology
University of Pennsylvania

Arthur L. Caplan

Center for Biomedical Ethics
University of Minnesota

Dan Farber

School of Law
University of Minnesota

Beth A. Fine

Graduate Program in Genetic
    Counseling
Northwestern University Medical
    School

Karen Grandstrand Gervais

Center for Biomedical Ethics
University of Minnesota
Minnesota Network of Institu-
    tional Ethics Committees

Phyllis Kahn

House of Representatives
State of Minnesota

Marc Lappé

Department of Medical
    Humanities
University of Illinois
College of Medicine

Bonnie S. LeRoy

Graduate Program in Genetic
    Counseling
Institute of Human Genetics
University of Minnesota

Joan H. Marks   Human Genetics Program
                                   Sarah Lawrence College

Walter E. Nance   Department of Human Genetics
                                   Medical College of Virginia
                                   Virginia Commonwealth
                                       University

Harry T. Orr   Department of Laboratory
                                       Medicine and Pathology
                                   Institute of Human Genetics
                                   University of Minnesota

James R. Sorenson   Department of Health Behavior
                                       and Health Education
                                   University of North Carolina

LeRoy Walters   Kennedy Institute of Ethics
                                   Georgetown University

Preface

Genetic counselors work at the intersection between the information produced by scientists and the hopes, dreams, and fears of clients whose lives could dramatically change as a result of receiving that information. Academic programs in genetic counseling were created to prepare professionals to assist physician and Ph.D. level geneticists to convey results of genetic testing and screening to clients. Considering that genetic counseling did not exist 20 years ago, the fact that the field is an accepted professional enterprise in universities, clinics, and hospitals throughout the United States is remarkable.

Ethical dilemmas facing genetic counselors, particularly with the advent of the Human Genome Project, are also remarkable. This volume is designed to place genetic counseling in the context of its history, current challenges, and future. Values are a central focus of our exploration. Questions addressed include: What are the central values that guide genetic counseling practice? Where did these values arise? Will current guiding values be relevant in the context of future options? What are the strengths and weaknesses of current approaches to client–counselor interaction? The goal of this examination is to illuminate the path on which genetic clients, counselors, policy makers, and our society will tread in the near future.

As a staff member of the Center for Biomedical Ethics, I first encountered clinical genetics when given an opportunity to teach in the Graduate Program in Genetic Counseling at the University of Minnesota. Journeying into the realm of genetic counselors and students has been fascinating, rewarding, and often challenging.

The task of learning enough of the language of genetics to converse with professionals conveyed some understanding of the complexity of transmitting genetic information in a meaningful way. Increasing familiarity with genetic conditions increased my sensitivity to the meaning and power this information could have in the lives of clients who receive it.

Counselors attempt to respond to client goals and questions while creating a supportive environment in which clients can begin to incorporate the results of genetic tests into the fabric of their lives and their decisions.

While exploring ethical concerns that arise in client–counselor interactions, I saw that the newly funded Human Genome Project will propel counselors through an even more challenging future course, one in which new gene marker mileposts appear almost daily (Orr, this volume). The nontechnological context of changing beliefs and values will also influence the evolution of the profession.

As an emerging profession, genetic counselors' beliefs and values reflect the dominant norms of the professionals who have provided counseling and the academic settings in which counseling usually occurs (Sorenson, this volume). Genetics and medicine rest on beliefs widely held in American society: that scientific progress is good and that highly sophisticated technologies are appropriate means to solving medical problems. The more understanding they gain about the nature and evolution of disease, the more prepared clinicians will be to treat, to ameliorate the effects, and to prevent future occurrence of disease.

A belief that medicine, including genetic medicine, is clear, factually based, and objective undergirds the strategies and norms of genetic counseling as well. Grounded in the assumption that facts and values are distinct entities, the counselor provides clear information regarding genetic conditions and available options. Nondirectiveness, a goal of counseling is meant to ensure that client rather than counselor values, determine how genetic information will influence health care decisions.

This nondirective stance also reflects the ethical principle of respect for client autonomy, which has taken priority over the principle of beneficence (acting in the patient's best interest) that had guided traditional medical practice. Legislation supporting the rights of patients to accept or refuse medical treatment paralleled the civil rights movement of the 1960s and early 1970s. Bioethicists added momentum to the shift in the balance of power from health care professional to client as the moral center for health care decision making.

Genetic counseling programs emerged in the midst of the evolution toward the concept of autonomy as a primary value. Counselors are particularly vigilant concerning client autonomy because of the private nature of reproductive decisions, and of the fact that genetic decisions often have major, long-term family consequences.

But client autonomy and the accompanying beliefs and values are being challenged on many fronts. Philosophers and social scientists question the validity of the fact/value distinction as a premise for client–professional interactions (Gervais, this volume). Some ethicists and policy makers identify the American emphasis on individualism, autonomy, and self-governance as major contributors to injustices that plague the health care system.

Across the spectrum of health care, professionals and policy makers are beginning to examine the level of autonomy consistent with social justice. For instance, how can the American health care system preserve the lives of thousands of unconscious elderly people and rescue the smallest infants while millions of citizens are without access to health care? Why are technologies being developed that make possible the creation of human embryos outside the body and their implantation into individuals who can afford this level of treatment, while many pregnant women and young children still experience the devastating effects of malnutrition and poverty? As a society we have come to recognize that difficult decisions must be made to distribute the burdens and benefits of health care responsibly.

In individual cases, conflicts occur when client and professional values differ. Professionals increasingly question their duty to grant all patient wishes. Families and professionals sometimes seek the intervention of courts of law to determine, for instance, whether to provide life-sustaining treatment to a permanently comatose patient.

Similar ethical challenges face genetic medicine and genetic counseling. On one hand, the Human Genome Project has been hailed as the Holy Grail of biology which will define what it is to be human and divulge the *cause* of a multitude of human problems. Alternatively, this technological quest is derided as the ultimate example of misapplied biological reductionism, which assumes that humans are the product of their genes alone.

> Unfortunately, it takes more than DNA to make a living organism . . . A living organism at any moment in its life is the unique consequence of a developmental history that results from the interaction of and determination by internal and external forces. The external forces, what we usually think of as 'environments,' are themselves partly a consequence of the activities of the organism itself as it produces and consumes the conditions of its own existence. Organisms do not find the world in which they develop. They make it. Reciprocally, the internal forces are not autonomous, but act in response to the external (Lewontin 1992).

Critics also dispute high-cost, high-technology approaches to human problems (including the Human Genome Project) because these endeavors divert funds that could be applied to solving social problems for those already afflicted by hunger, homelessness, illness, and discrimination. The ability to identify many individuals affected by genetic conditions raises major medical and social concerns regarding which tests will be made available, to whom they will be offered, how testing will be paid for, and which decisions will be made as a result of the tests. George

Annas cites the proposal for universal cystic fibrosis screening, which is a current subject of debate among professionals.

> Should prenatal cystic fibrosis screening be made available to every woman in the United States, as has been suggested by many? The cost is not trivial. Assuming half of the pregnant women in the United States got this test at a cost of $100, it would cost $200 million a year—the entire genome budget. So it is not the money that is spent on building the human genome's infrastructure that should have us thinking, but the money that will be spent on each and every test that comes out of the human genome project. Again, the question is should we be putting our money in developing tests that only relatively well-to-do individuals can take advantage of? (Annas 1992)

Most genetic counseling clients are middle and upper middle class, highly educated individuals who have sufficient insurance and/or finances to cover the costs of testing. Couples seeking counseling share values with the professionals from whom they seek help; these couples believe it is their right, if not their responsibility, to control personal reproductive decisions. These shared perceptions may not be relevant for people with other backgrounds, who hold alternative views of illness, disease, and the relationship of individuals to society.

Whether the Human Genome Project will be an agent of salvation from medical problems or a tool to further the goals of an elitist society is yet undecided. But whatever the outcome, the advent of the project with its potential for genetic information and biological control is compelling a reexamination of basic understandings of the goals of medicine and the processes of client–practitioner communication.

Ethical dilemmas facing genetic counselors today will challenge primary practitioners in the near future when genetic information becomes more accessible. Resolution of some counseling issues may provide a prototype for broader social consideration of genetic technologies in the future: Is nondirectiveness really possible? Should individual autonomy take precedence over the needs of others? Should practitioners inform individuals of an available test not covered by insurance? How can statistical probabilities be made meaningful for health care decision making? What about providing gender information so clients can consider terminating a pregnancy if the child is the *wrong* sex? How can professional autonomy and the dictates of personal conscience be incorporated into the counseling process?

As genetic possibilities become realities, it is imperative that professionals, clients, policy makers, and the general public scrutinize the values inherent in the health care system and the social and ethical consequences of communicating genetic information. Focus on values that do guide and ought to guide genetic counseling is meant to provoke introspection on the part of the reader. We hope that this examination can also serve as a foundation from which to begin to address some legal, ethical, and policy considerations in the expanding universe of clinical genetics, one that will profoundly affect the future of us all.

Dianne M. Bartels

Introduction

Discussions about the role of genetic counseling in the future assume that the Human Genome Project will pose significant new challenges. For readers who are unfamiliar with them, this overview provides a basic description of the Human Genome Project and of some challenges that are likely to emerge with developing genetic technologies.

Genetics in Medicine

The science of genetics first became a tool for medicine in the 1950s when chromosome abnormalities were determined to have a major role in malformation, retardation, infertility, and reproductive failure. This discovery brought genetic problems into the realm of clinical medicine (Thompson 1986). Since the middle of the 1970s, powerful new molecular genetic technologies have allowed practitioners to analyze human hereditary material. Using chromosome tests and gene markers for specific diseases, geneticists can identify persons with inheritable conditions and identify carriers, individuals who although unaffected themselves, carry genes that may be inherited by future generations. New technologies also permit physicians to do presymptomatic testing; that is, to identify persons who will be affected by a genetic condition prior to the time they develop symptoms.

Overview of the Human Genome Project

Objectives and Scope

The Human Genome Project will hasten the development of genetic technologies. The mission of the project is to identify the full set of inherited instructions contained inside our cells and to read the complete genetic text that makes up the hereditary material. The goal of this international effort is to provide scientists with new tools to help them understand the molecular essence of devastating human illnesses such as cancer, schizophrenia, and Alzheimers disease. The project will attempt to determine how environmental factors and gene defects contribute to the development of common disorders such as heart disease, diabetes, immune disorders, and birth defects (NCHGR, 1990).

The Human Genome Project has two major components. The first and primary contribution of the project will be the development of chromosome maps that are diagrams to help scientists locate specific genes responsible for determining particular human traits. Scientists will develop two kinds of maps. First, researchers will develop linkage maps by studying the location of disease genes in the genome to better understand the way diseases are inherited in families. These maps are created utilizing blood samples from several generations of family members where some are affected by a genetic condition. The second kind of chromosome map is called a physical map. This tool allows researchers to identify the actual arrangement and distances between genes on a chromosome. Having a detailed genetic map enables scientists to understand the structure of genes and to characterize the molecular defects that result in genetic problems.

The second major component of the Human Genome Project is called DNA sequencing. Once the genes have been located on a map, the next goal is to determine the sequence of the chemical, DNA, in each gene. The order of bases that make up our genetic material determines the information carried by genes. Genes instruct cells to make proteins by the assembling of amino acids, the building blocks of proteins. The amino acids must be assembled in precisely the correct order for a protein to function properly. Otherwise, the protein building process may be disrupted and the protein that is produced will be unable to perform its function. For example, sickle cell anemia results when a protein in red blood cells is assembled with one incorrect amino acid in the chain. The resulting change in the solubility of the cell's hemoglobin causes the cells to sickle leading to serious tissue damage, severe illness, and sometimes death.

Analysis of the information produced by gene maps and DNA sequencing will revolutionize our understanding of how genes control the function of the human body. Detailed maps will help scientists find and study the genes involved in a variety of human diseases. This new knowledge will facilitate the development of new clinical strategies to prevent, diagnose, and treat human diseases (NCHGR 1990).

Project Funding

In 1988, the United States Congress appropriated funds specifically for this human genetics research effort. The dollar amount allotted has increased from $17.2 million in 1988 to $87 million in 1991. When the U.S. Human Genome Project is functioning at full capacity, it will require an estimated $200 million each year to operate. These appropriations will be shared by the National Center for Human Genome Research (NCHGR) and the U.S. Department of Energy (DOE), which has an independently managed human genome program. The NCHGR administers all National Institutes of Health (NIH) research funds dedicated to these efforts. The NIH Program Advisory Committee is composed of scientific experts from industry, academia, and non-profit corporations who offer guidance on the strategy and direction of NCHGR-supported research.

Beginning in 1990, NCHGR made an unprecedented commitment to fund a program designed to address ethical, legal, and social questions arising out of this effort to map and explain the role of genetic material predictive of adverse health outcomes. For the first time basic scientists, legal experts, philosophers, health care professionals, social scientists, and consumers are discussing the future social implications of a field of scientific research. A significant portion of the 1992 funds for the Human Genome Project—5% of the NIH contribution and 3% of the DOE contribution—is dedicated to studying the implications of human genome research. To date, this is the largest United States investment in ethical, legal, and social analysis of emerging technologies.

Ethical Challenges in Genetic Testing

The following discussion identifies some of the major social and ethical issues that are likely to confront policy makers and the public in response to developments made possible by the Human Genome Project.

Discrimination/Fairness

Genetic test results that identify pre-existing medical conditions may be the basis for the denial of insurance coverage (Farber, Kahn this volume). Life, health, and disability insurance carriers can use results of genetic screening to increase the rates for individuals with genetic conditions that are costly to manage. Furthermore, companies could deny or limit coverage to healthy people in whom genetic tests predict the future occurrence of a genetic condition. Within the workplace, genetic screening test results may be used to detect workers with susceptibilities to harmful effects of occupational exposures. Many insurance companies and employers are considering the advisability of mandatory screening for diseases relevant to risk status or fitness for a particular job.

America's history with genetic testing to identify sickle cell disease in the in the early 1960s counsels caution in this age of human genome research. Sickle cell anemia is an inherited disorder that is found in a relatively circumscribed population that includes African Americans and individuals who come from Mediterranean areas. Public health measures to screen all African American children for sickle cell anemia were not accompanied by appropriate public education campaigns. One author described the program and its tragic consequences as follows:

> What went wrong? The sickle cell program was launched with the best of intentions and a great deal of zeal—perhaps too much zeal. Some states even passed laws requiring testing of newborns, school children, marriage license applicants, and prison inmates. But far too little thought—and too few resources—were devoted to education and counseling to see that people understood the information they were being given.
>
> The upshot is that screening engendered tremendous confusion and anxiety. Many of those identified as carriers mistakenly thought they were afflicted with this debilitating disease. All too often, confidentiality was breached, and in some cases, carriers were stigmatized and denied health insurance.
>
> At the time, no prenatal test was available, and some carriers were told that the only way to prevent the disease was to avoid having children. This message, coming from outside the black community, led to charges of racism. (Roberts, 1990)

One of the fundamental goals of the genetic counseling profession is to educate counselors to serve as public educators and advocates for persons affected by genetic conditions so such travesties can be avoided in the future.

Privacy/Confidentiality

Clinics, laboratories, counselors, and health care systems will need to develop systems to protect the privacy of genetic information they gather. Commercial testing done in private laboratories raises concerns about the confidentiality and uses of data acquired without documentation and protection by laws limiting access to public medical records. Calls for mandatory genetic screening raise the question of how a vast data bank of personal information on all members of society will be protected from misuse.

Personal Health/Lifestyle Testing

With an increasing ability to detect genetic conditions prior to symptom development, information about health maintenance and disease prevention will be available to those who seek it. When genetic screens become a routine part of medical examinations, it is likely that individuals will be expected to utilize the information as part of personal health maintenance. Will policy makers share those expectations and will insurers base decisions about coverage of health care costs on the degree of responsibility an individual has exerted to ameliorate or prevent predictable genetic symptoms? Will responsible citizens be expected to avail themselves of opportunities for genetic screening?

Resource Allocation

Genetic counseling today is sought primarily by upper middle class, highly educated people. New knowledge will increase the alternatives available and the demand for genetic counseling and treatment services. With a recognition that universal screening programs could decrease the number of people with genetic problems in the health care system, public health and financial concerns may create expectations that such screening programs become routine. As universal screening programs expand, the current supply of health care professionals providing genetic counseling will not be sufficient to meet future needs. To extend services to a more diverse client population will require new mechanisms to make them available and to pay for these services.

Genetic Counseling and the Human Genome Project

This book focuses primarily on challenges in genetic client-counselor interactions. To address ethical considerations in individual cases, it is always important to recognize that these relationships occur in a larger context. Technological advances and changing societal values will continue to influence genetic counseling practices. Conversely, genetic counseling professionals can contribute to better policy outcomes by sharing relevant features of what they learn in practice.

Elizabeth Truesdell-Smith
Dianne M. Bartels

Acknowledgments

A cast of contributors has made publication of this volume possible. We first want to thank the chapter authors, whose scholarship defines the substance of this analysis of genetic counseling. Authors were willing not only to share their expertise, but to interact with other authors and expand their manuscripts based on that dialogue.

We are grateful for financial support from the National Center for Human Genome Research, which allowed us to actualize our vision and complete the work of this project. Eric Juengst, Acting Chief of the Ethical, Legal, and Social Implications (ELSI branch) program, has been an inspirational advisor providing both intellectual and moral support.

Michael Yesley, Co-ordinator, Department of Energy, ELSI Program, participated in the initial conference from which this volume is derived, and hosted a meeting providing an opportunity to share information and receive feedback from other grant recipients and ELSI members.

Anthony Faras, Director of the Institute of Human Genetics, created the foundation for this discussion by supporting the development of the Graduate Program in Genetic Counseling at the University of Minnesota.

Elizabeth Truesdell-Smith organized references for the initial meeting, recorded the proceedings, and completed a summary reading packet describing ethical issues related to genetic testing and screening. Her positive approach, organizational ability, and unfailing patience and warmth made the process of creating this book almost a joy.

Toni Knezevich revised this mansucript for submission. Her energy, competence, kindness, and humor are daily sources of support in the University of Minnesota's Center for Biomedical Ethics.

We are deeply grateful for this opportunity to learn all that we have about genetic counseling and for the continuing support that allows us to share what we have learned.

Dianne M. Bartels, Bonnie S. LeRoy, and
Arthur L. Caplan

PART I

Evolution of Genetic Counseling

Chapter 1

Genetic Counseling: Values That Have Mattered

JAMES R. SORENSON

Introduction

The title of this chapter is "Genetic Counseling: Values That Have Mattered." It will address three issues:

1. The transition of genetic counseling from eugenics to medical genetics;
2. The origins and applications of 'value neutrality' in genetic counseling; and,
3. The range of values that have guided genetic counseling in the United States.

Before addressing these issues, however, I would like to put my comments in perspective. First, concerning the concept of 'value neutrality,' my bias is that genetic counseling as an applied activity can not be value neutral. To apply knowledge requires making decisions about what to inform people, when to inform them, and how to inform them. These decisions are influenced by values, and in this respect, genetic counseling probably has never been nor ever will be value neutral. I think the issue that is of more interest for genetic counseling is the value of "nondirectiveness."

Second, I will attempt to identify some of the major values, in addition to "nondirectiveness," that have guided genetic counseling over its more recent history. In this analysis it is important to recognize that genetic counseling in this country is not a distinct full-fledged profession in a sociological sense. Hence, it is difficult to speak of genetic counseling as a

3

unified enterprise. More accurately, genetic counseling has been and is a consulting activity that has been and continues to be practiced by a variety of professionals. Understanding the various professional groups and their organizational and institutional settings is useful in appreciating the evolution and the particular value profile of genetic counseling in the United States.

Finally, for purposes of gaining insight into genetic counseling as a consulting activity, I would like to suggest that it is useful to identify three phases in its development in this country. These are (1) the period from the late 1800s to the late 1930s, (2) the period from the late 1930s to the late 1960s, and (3) the period from the late 1960s until today. I have identified four topics that allow some comparison of similarities and differences in genetic counseling during these periods. These are (1) the providers/ practitioners of genetic counseling, (2) the organizational and institutional settings of counseling, (3) genetic counseling clients, and finally (4) the goals and objectives of counseling. I do not maintain that these are the only phases one could identify, nor the only set of factors on which to compare these or other phases. Rather, I have found them useful in thinking about the evolution of genetic counseling as a type of consulting activity.

Eugenics and Genetic Counseling

The first period from the late 1800s to the late 1930s constitutes the major period of the eugenics era in this country (Ludmerer 1972). In abbreviated form the practitioners of eugenics were largely self pro-claimed experts in social reform—including clinical psychologists, staffs of mental institutions, an assortment of academics, primarily biologists and social scientists, but interestingly comparatively few physicians. The organizational setting of applied genetics in this era involved various organizations including the old Eugenics Record Office in Cold Spring Harbor, NY, as well as other private and voluntary organizations. Institu-tionally, genetics during this period was applied primarily through the state and federal government, with the passage of laws concerning immi-gration, marriage, procreation, and the institutionalization of people deemed "unfit" to reproduce or be on their own.

Of particular importance in understanding the nature of the eugenics era is the fact that applied human genetics generally, and genetic counsel-ing in particular, was part of a social movement. As such, the eugenics movement provided both a mission and a method for applied genetics. The mission was, as I have commented elsewhere:

both Arcadian as well as Utopian. It was Arcadian to the extent that many within the movement looked to the past as an ideal and they were attempting to reconstruct an assumed lost purity of the American race, or to recapture the simplicity of an earlier form of social existence. The movement was also Utopian in that it looked to the future as an opportunity to improve men and society, through selective breeding, immigration, and social planning. In both its Arcadian dreams and Utopian fantasies it looked to genetics as the method. (Sorenson 1976)

This philosophic dualism is one premise of the application of genetics that has undergone revision and, in fact, has been rejected as applied genetics has evolved during the past 60 years in this country.

The recipients or clients of genetic services during this first era, if such terms are appropriate, were usually not those seeking eugenic measures but rather individuals identified by the state as needing procreative regulation or regulation of citizenship.

Lastly, the goals and objectives of the eugenics era encompassed biological as well as social ends. The biological goals revolved about the preservation and purification of the race or biological stock of the nation. Socially there was the objective of reducing the social and economic burden on society of those deemed biologically and/or socially "unfit."

The eugenics era witnessed a highly coercive approach to applied human genetics. Genetic counseling was part of this initiative, but probably not a large part. While the evidence is limited, one can surmise that nondirective counseling was not a mainstay of genetic counseling offered during this period. The state, through the passage of laws and immigration policies, among other initiatives, was a major vehicle for enforcement and regulation. What is clear is that the goals and objectives of applied genetics, including genetic counseling, were stated, most often, in terms of population-based social/biological criteria. And although there was no single professional group defining the goals or objectives of genetic counseling, there was considerable social support for such goals and objects fostered by a social movement.

From Eugenics to Clinical Medicine

The next "phase" of genetic counseling covers the period from the late 1930s through the late 1960s. One can ask if there was a link between genetic counseling in the eugenics era and its characteristics in the period from the mid-1930s through the late 1960s. There is some difference of opinion on this. Let me quote two sources. Wertz and Fletcher, in a recent commentary on the history of genetic counseling in the United States, wrote "There was no historical continuity between the eugenics movement. . . . and the new field of human genetics and genetic counseling that began to develop before and especially after WWI" (Wertz and Fletcher 1989). Citing the writing of Sheldon Reed, they note a significant difference in the place of nondirective counseling in the newer era in contrast to the eugenic era.

A contrary position is adopted by Ludmerer, who, in his history of applied human genetics (written in the early 1970s) in the United States, stated, "Today's heredity clinics . . . descended directly from the early eugenics movement. Eugenic thought, in a precise, unpretentious form, had survived the original movement. Eugenics has divorced itself from Spencerian sociology and entered medicine" (Ludmerer 1972).

During this second phase there were two major developments. First there was the demise of the eugenics movement, well chronicled elsewhere. Second, there was the movement of genetic counseling out of the organizational and institutional context of the eugenics movement into academia, including the academic medical world.

In some respects one could divide this latter period into two subphases. The first focuses on the emergence of genetic counseling largely in the scholarly academic world, following the demise of the eugenics era. Second, beginning in the mid- to late 1940s, applied human genetics began to make its way into the medical world, through the emergence of departments of medical and clinical genetics in a few and then more medical schools around the country.

If one focuses during this era on the application of genetics in the academic world, especially during the early period, it is possible to develop the impression that there was some linkage between genetic counseling in the eugenics era and this newer period. For example, the writings of some academic geneticists during this period reflect a lingering concern about the population implications of genetic counseling. On the other hand, if one focuses on genetic counseling during the later part of this period, when it was becoming strongly entrenched in academic medicine, one would get the impression that genetic counseling bore much less resemblance to its eugenic predecessor, since concern with the population impact of genetic counseling lost virtually all favor among clinically oriented medical geneticists.

In terms of practitioners during this phase, in the early period they tended to be Ph.D. academic-based geneticists, often in biology or zoology departments in universities. It may be overdrawing the case somewhat, but this generation of genetic counselors practiced genetic counseling, one might say, almost by accident. What I mean is that they had expertise in genetics, as it was developing then, and when reproductive problems involving suspected genetic factors occurred they were about the only ones available who could provide some information. They did not view genetic counseling as a professional calling.

In the mid to latter part of this phase genetic counseling began a significant movement into the medical world. While trained in medicine, a group of academic physicians, not unlike their counterparts in the more liberal arts academic world (Ph.D.s), practiced genetic counseling "accidentally," that is, more because they happened to be experts in a developing and esoteric body of knowledge than because of a specific calling or commitment to the practical application of genetic knowledge. As such, both Ph.D.s and early M.D. geneticists were, one might argue, more "scholarly" than "consulting" professionals. Why might this be important?

Eliot Freidson, a medical sociologist, has argued that there are important differences between the orientation of scholars regarding the use and application of their expertise and the orientation of "practitioners" or, as he would label them, consulting professionals (Freidson, 1970). One of the key differences is that the scholarly oriented professionals tend to view their obligation toward the use of their expertise as largely one of presenting the facts and information. The user makes the decision as to what to do with the knowledge. How the information is used is generally viewed as outside the technical and scientific competence of the scholarly professional. As such, Freidson argues that scholars tend to maintain an "ideology of technical neutrality" regarding the use of their expertise.

In contrast, consulting professionals, according to Freidson, tend to view their role in the application of their expertise in a more activist, interventionist position. By the very nature of their training, often with significant clinical experience, consulting professionals become accustomed to, and in fact expect to be participants in decisions about the use of their expertise. They develop what Freidson calls a sense of "functionally diffuse wisdom" in contrast to an ideology of value neutrality. By functionally diffuse wisdom Freidson is not attempting to put down practitioners. Rather the point he is making is that in the process of dealing with recurring human dilemmas and problems practitioners come to believe that they have special insight into human nature. This special insight "equips" practitioners to believe they should advise and intervene in other peoples' lives. This belief translates into a willingness to offer advice and counsel on practical matters, often matters on which the professional has no special training or technical expertise.

I am suggesting that one of the factors contributing to the origins of a nondirective value in genetic counseling may have developed in part because of the "scholarly" orientation and role definition of the first set of genetic counselors following the eugenics era. Certainly academic Ph.Ds., but also academic physicians in academic medical centers were, by their training and orientation, oriented more to the scholarly development of new knowledge and understanding of the world than to the day-to-day practical application of their expertise and the solution of problems. As such, their professional orientation would make them more likely to exercise "value neutrality" than "functionally diffuse wisdom" in the application of their expertise, to be nondirective in philosophy and practice.

An additional factor in understanding the delivery of genetic counseling in this phase is its organizational and institutional settings. Genetic counseling had left the voluntary organization and social movement context of the eugenics era and entered largely, but not exclusively, academia and medical research organizations. In such settings, in contrast to the eugenics era, there was little by way of institutional support for or concern with the "eugenic" or social implications of and potential for eugenic measures. Eugenics was being rapidly discredited, as Ludmerer has noted, both in terms of its scientific base and in terms of its political acceptability (Ludmerer 1972). Additionally, with the movement of genetic counseling into the medical arena there was a pronounced diminution of interest in the social implications of the application of such knowledge in contrast to its potential utility in assisting the individual client or patient. In short, with the movement of genetic expertise into institutional medicine there was no longer significant institutional support for considering the social implications of the application of such knowledge. The delivery of genetic counseling by more academic than consulting professionals contributed to an emphasis in genetic counseling on education more than counseling.

The recipients/clients of genetic counseling in this phase, in large part, were individuals who were referred to genetic experts because of previous genetic based or influenced reproductive problems. Whether they acted on the information provided by their "genetic counselors" or other family counselors, the clients in this period were beginning to make decisions regarding whether they wanted to have and use such information. In large part they obtained genetic counseling through care of their affected infant or child in a specialty clinic or because of the family physician's awareness of the potential utility of seeing someone with more expertise than they in genetics.

To assess the goals and objectives of the practitioners during this phase one has to look at the writings of numerous genetic counselors. Dr. Sheldon Reed clearly advocated a nondirective approach to counseling and by implication suggested that the primary goal of genetic counseling was education. Reed is credited with selecting genetic counseling as the name of this activity (Reed 1955). However, as noted above, if one examines the writings of other experts, such as Herndon, Dice, and Stern, there was an undercurrent of discussion in their writing suggesting that in providing genetic counseling the provider should be aware of the possible negative eugenic, or population implications of counseling (Haller 1963; Ludmerer 1972). Such statements were usually quickly followed by discussion of two sets of considerations. The first was that the decisions about what to do reproductively could not be informed or made by counselors because they did not have the expertise to inform such a decision and second, usually they did not know the patient/client and his/her situation well enough to offer advice. The writings of providers during this era suggested a strong faith in the clients to make a wise choice, or, in the language of today, a more informed reproductive decision. Translated, this meant that knowledge of an elevated risk would lead more often than not to decisions not to have a (another) child, and hence, the negative eugenic implications of genetic counseling would be limited. This faith, or assumption, was perhaps grounded less in concerns about the eugenic impact of genetic counseling than faith in the role of knowledge in human affairs, a not uncommon belief among scholarly optimists as opposed to the sometimes pessimistic views of consulting professionals.

The Professionalization of Genetic Counseling

The next phase, from the late 1960s to today, is a particularly important period of development for genetic counseling. This era witnessed the first institutional attempts to define genetic counseling (Fraser 1974), the development of the first training programs in this country targeted explicitly for the preparation of genetic counselors, and the development of certification of counselors (Kenen 1984). Moreover, it was during this period that developments in clinical genetics, including heterozygote screening for Tay–Sachs and sickle cell carrier status emerged, as did prenatal diagnosis for a variety of genetic/chromosomal disorders. It was also a period when some of the initial reports began to appear on the effects of genetic counseling on reproductive behavior.

Looking first at the providers of counseling, during this period counseling continued its movement into the medical arena from liberal arts. A survey in the early 1970s suggested that the majority of practitioners were M.D.s working in tertiary care settings (Sorenson and Culbert 1977). The provision of genetic counseling by these research-physicians is significant because it maintained the provisions of counseling by professionals who, in many ways, were more scholarly than consulting in their orientation. This reinforced, to some degree, the initial orientation of counseling in terms of its nondirective orientation and reinforced the emphasis on genetic counseling more as an educational than a counseling activity.

While tertiary care medical genetic professionals remain a very significant component of counseling, this phase witnessed the development of a special group of masters level prepared genetic counselors, genetic associates, and even the training of laypeople to provide counseling, usually associated with sickle cell trait screening programs.

Kenen (1984) chronicled the development of masters level genetic counselors in this country. An examination of the curricula of most genetic associate training programs suggests that their orientation seems to be modeled largely on that of the physicians with whom they collaborate in the provision of counseling. This means that the primary preparation of this group of new professionals is on the provision of technical medical and especially genetic information, with there being comparatively limited attention to the practice of specific patient–client counseling strategies. What is clear is that this professional group, as a whole, endorsed a nondirective posture toward genetic counseling in their code of ethics.

Near the end of this era, usually as part of prenatal diagnosis, genetic counseling began to be incorporated into more routine primary care, especially obstetrics and gynecology. Medical schools began to incorporate expanded genetics offerings in curricula. This is significant, because it signals the beginnings of genetic counseling being provided not only by tertiary care physicians and genetic counselors, but by primary care-oriented physicians as well. Following the scholarly versus consulting distinction introduced above, this development would suggest that in the hands of primary care physicians, having perhaps more of a "functionally diffuse wisdom" ethic than "value neutrality" orientation, counseling could become more directive than when practiced by tertiary care provides.

A collorary to the increasing number of types of professionals providing counseling has been growth in the organizational and institutional settings in which counseling is provided. Expanding out from academic medical centers, genetic counseling as part of genetic screening programs has increased its presence in public health settings. This expansion brought with it, in addition to newborn genetic disease screening, the development of trait screening programs (sickle cell and Tay–Sachs), and the use of legislation to promulgate such screening, especially sickle cell trait screening programs (National Academy of Sciences, 1975). Since this experience, often negative, there has been a significant backing away from such legislative initiatives.

During this period there has been an expansion in the number of types of individuals receiving genetic counseling. Whereas during the early phases of this period probably most individuals receiving counseling did so because of a known reproductive problem in their family, increasingly, especially through genetic trait screening programs, as well as prenatal diagnosis, people began being counseled who had no reason to suspect that they were at any special or unusual risk to have a child with a birth defect or specific genetic problem.

The goals of genetic counseling have been only somewhat altered during this era. In contrast to Kessler, I do not think there has been, to any large degree, a paradigm shift from preventive medicine to psychological counseling during this era (Kessler 1980). What there has been, especially during the mid part of this period, was (1) recognition of the psychological complexity of counseling, if one took the concept of counseling seriously, and (2) a broadening of the focus of various evaluation studies from examining reproductive outcomes in terms of risk magnitude and estimated burdensomeness of a genetic disorder, to an examination of additional determinates of reproductive decisions, including the desire to have a child, family circumstances, and other psychosocial factors (Frets and Niermeyer 1990). Such research has suggested the complexity of client reproductive decision making and the difficulties that the provision of effective counseling, as opposed to genetic education, would entail.

Conclusions

Genetic counseling will continue to evolve, spurred on by its own unique history as well as by practical developments resulting from the human genome initiative. Before looking ahead, however, I would like to summarize a few major points concerning the value of nondirectiveness as well as identify other values that have shaped genetic counseling during the past 60 years.

The origins of nondirectiveness in genetic counseling reside, I believe, to a significant degree in the institutional settings that counseling found itself in subsequent to the eugenics movement, and especially in the types of professionals who provided this service. It is also the case that reaction to the abuses of the eugenics movement must have conditioned virtually all practitioners to be cautious about too willingly offering advice or directly instructing clients as to what were good or bad reproductive decisions. I would also argue that genetic counseling has been, and remains in large part misnamed. While recognizing both the difficulties that Reed faced in selecting a name for this activity decades ago, as well as attempts by various training programs to bring more counseling into genetic counseling since then, I think the weight of evidence suggests that the label of "genetic consult" more aptly describes what usually transpires in "genetic counseling." Recognizing the psychosocial complexity of the issues genetic counseling can raise for clients and the usual practical arrangement of one or at most two client visits with some follow-up telephone calls, there usually is little counseling, a time-consuming activity requiring training that is rarely in the experience of most physicians offering this service, and only slightly more in the training of genetic counselors.

In addition to valuing nondirectiveness over advice giving and education over counseling, I think that one can identify four additional values shaping the practice of genetic counseling over the past several decades. First, making (more) informed reproductive decisions has been considered better than making less informed decisions. Setting aside the difficult issue of what knowledge makes a reproductive decision more informed, the entire genetic counseling enterprise is predicated on the belief that an informed decision is better than a less informed one.

A second value has been that the primary focus of genetic counseling is the individual or couple, more so than the community or society. This value reflects in large part the institutional pressure in medicine to focus on the individual and view the delivery of services and their justification more from the perspective of the individual than society.

A third value has been that the effectiveness of genetic counseling resides more in its utility to individuals and couples confronted with reproductive risks than to a reduction of birth defects in at-risk populations. Although there is some interest in the latter, an examination of studies assessing the effectiveness of genetic counseling demonstrates that virtually all of these have focused on client knowledge acquisition in counseling, with much less attention given to the psychological adjustment of clients, and very little attention given to changes in the rates of infants born with birth defects in high-risk groups. Even when the latter has been reported, it is often noted that the real measure of successful counseling resides in clients making more informed decisions. To the degree that genetic counseling has embraced the philosophy and values of preventive medicine, it would appear that there is much more concern with the prevention of uninformed reproductive decisions than in the prevention of birth defects.

Finally, another value in genetic counseling to date has been its predominant focus on phenotypic, not genotypic variation. Stated differently, an examination of clinical genetic counseling texts shows that attention is given to discussing risks for phenotypically describable disease states, much more so than genotypic carrier states. Parallel to this, while it is increasingly possible to identify genotypic variation using prenatal diagnosis, screening for such purposes is normally frowned on. Genetic screening programs specifically targeting the identification of carriers might appear to be at variance with this. However, even here it seems that the primary emphasis is on enabling two carriers to make a more informed reproductive decision, more so than developing programs that would focus on carrier status.

Genetic Counseling in the Future

Turning from the past to the near future, it would appear that many of the values identified above will continue to play a major role in the delivery of genetic counseling. It is possible, as noted above, that as genetic counseling is delivered by primary care physicians it could become more directive.

During its history, and still today, genetic counseling has focused primarily on the provision of information useful for making reproductive decisions. Although this will continue to be the case, it is possible that genetic counseling may expand its focus to include other types of "counseling," for example, life-style, education, and counseling. The reason for this lies in research, some of it conducted before the human genome initiative, but some of it growing directly out of this massive scientific enterprise. For example, it is increasingly possible to identify "genetic markers" for susceptibility to certain types of chronic diseases, such as various forms of cardiovascular disease, diabetes, and cancer. Armed with such information it increasingly will be possible to identify individuals at an elevated risk for developing such diseases and to counsel them on specific dietary and other life-style factors as well as screening procedures that they could use to reduce their risk. Counseling to reduce the risks of such diseases has grown dramatically in this and other countries, spurred on generally by the health promotion and disease prevention movement of the past decade (Becker and Rosenstock 1989). But such counseling, usually provided by health educators and delivered in medical as well as public health settings, has focused almost exclusively on behaviorally based risk factors, such as smoking, lack of exercise, and excessive drinking. There is increasingly genetic risk counseling, usually for selected genetic based cancer and cardiovascular diseases (Lerman, Rimer, and Engstrom 1991). Should genetic counseling begin to incorporate such counseling on a large basis it will expand its focus to include not only reproductive counseling, but health promotion and disease prevention counseling as well. This would be a dramatic new phase in the evolution of "genetic counseling."

Genetic counseling over its past 60 years has lost, to a great extent, both its Arcadian dreams as well as Utopian fantasies of a biologically pure and socially perfect world. In the place of such global and abstract goals has been placed the more limited objective of helping clients make more informed reproductive decisions. With the advent of the Human Genome Project and the projection of a much broader application of applied human genetics in society there is increasing debate about the appropriate use of existing and new genetic knowledge. Genetic counseling should be included as part of this debate (Tables 1-3).

Table 1.   Three Phases in the Development of Genetic Counseling in the
United States

Phases			
A	*B*	*C*	*D*
Late 1800s–	*Late 1930s–*	*Late 1960s–*	*1991–2000*
Late 1930s	*Late 1960s*	*Late 1991s*	

*a*Comparison bases: (1) providers/practicitioners; (2) organizational/institutional
settings; (3) clients; (4) goals/objectives.

Table 2.   Factors Contributing to the Development of a Norm of Value
Neutrality (Nondirectiveness) in Genetic Counseling

1. Discrediting of eugenic biological and social ideas, scientifically, and politically.
2. Movement of genetic counseling into institutional settings (academia and academic medicine) that did not support, generally, collective (societal) justifications for the coercive practical application of expertise.
3. Provision of genetic counseling, subsequent to the eugenics era, more by "scholarly" than by "consulting" professionals.
4. Evolving definition of genetic counseling more as an educational than a eugenic/preventive medicine intiative, first by key spokespeople, then institutionally.
5. Evaluation studies suggesting that the calculus of decision making is influenced less than anticipated by risk magnitude/disease burden consideration than by a combination of social/psychological factors.

Table 3.   Major Values Guiding Genetic Counseling in the United States

1. Informed reproductive decision making is better than less/noninformed decision making.
2. Nondirective counseling is preferable to directive counseling.
3. A primary goal of genetic counsling is the provision of information, more so than assisting counselees in making a decision.
4. The primary focus or unit of analysis and intervention is the individual and possibly the family, but not society.
5. Although there is an interest in the biological impact of genetic counseling, this is assessed by looking at the occurrence of disease in a family, and their ability to cope with such problems, more so than at an aggregate/population level, either phenotypically or genotypically.

Chapter 2

The Training of Genetic Counselors: Origins of a Psychosocial Model

JOAN H. MARKS

Sheldon Reed is universally credited as the author of the term genetic counseling. However, a detailed review of the literature reveals only scant documentation of the term's origin. In a 1947 publication Dr. Reed suggested that the term genetic counseling was preferable to the then current terms that included genetic advice or genetic hygiene. He described genetic counseling as "a kind of social work done for the benefit of the whole family entirely without eugenic connotations" (Reed 1963). The profession of Genetic Counseling initiated in 1969 has in fact, evolved according to the concept suggested by Reed in 1947 (Marks and Richter 1974).

The purpose of this volume, as I see it, is to review the responsibilities of genetic counselors as we prepare for a future in which increasing numbers of genetically determined disorders will be identified and mapped to specific genes, thus opening new, albeit more complex challenges for the genetic counselor. Therefore, I feel I can best contribute to this purpose by reviewing the evolution and curriculum of the first program to train genetic counselors.

Genetic counseling is a relatively new health profession. The first formal masters level program to train genetic counselors was initiated only 22 years ago. The challenge in training genetic counselors was then, and continues to be, one of providing an adequate, sound biological curriculum, while also emphasizing the importance of training in psychological counseling. Training programs also address the broader, if somewhat less well defined, ethical and societal issues that we now recognize are integral to genetic counseling.

15

Mapping the human genome will lead to the identification of genes responsible for genetic disorders for which specific markers have not previously been available. In addition, mapping the human genome will lead to recognition of genes that place individuals at risk for various disorders. For example, the potential for identifying individuals at risk for conditions such as cancer, where prevention or early intervention is important, may become a major new dimension of genetic counseling. In this context the Human Genome Project will expand the traditional areas for genetic counseling. Those of us responsible for the curriculum for genetic counselors should realize that the current understanding of the genetic basis of disease necessarily expands the requirements for the training of genetic counselors. The requirements of the future, therefore, underscore the appropriateness of examining the current status of genetic counseling practices today.

In addition to describing the origins and evolution of training for genetic counselors, I will address the issue of value neutrality as it relates to the training of counselors.

An Underserved Population: Families with Genetic Disease

In 1968 when Melissa L. Richter, a member of the Sarah Lawrence biology faculty, began to examine the field of human genetics with the idea of developing a training program at Sarah Lawrence, she wrote in a memo to the Dean of the college:

> The need for genetic counseling is far greater than the services available today; more families carry inherited disease than can be adequately diagnosed and counseled by the handful of physicians trained in human genetics. Moreover, most patients who do receive counseling are selected not because of their need but because they have the illness that fits the research interests of the physician in question. The best genetic counselors state that there is a demand for diagnosing and counseling in human genetics they cannot meet. Few medical schools give training in the specialty of human genetics, and no graduate schools specifically train counselors for this medical profession. The dearth of adequate medical counseling is particularly sad. Persons with inherited diseases now represent a larger proportion of the patients in this country than ever before (700 babies a day with inherited defects). Of the hundreds of thousands in this country who have manifestations of inherited disease, few can find counseling to determine the exact nature and the exact mode of inheritance of the disease, or the probability of transmitting it to their offspring. Most go uninformed and unguided. Very few apparently healthy people ever have medical examinations to detect a genetic disease for which they might be a carrier. (Richter 1968)

This prescient statement persuaded Sarah Lawrence to initiate a master's level program. It is my impression that the need recognized 22 years ago is still with us today, and will probably be even greater in the future.

Physicians prominent in medical genetics encouraged Sarah Lawrence to proceed swiftly with the proposed training program. Among them were highly respected physicians and counselors in human genetics, Dr. Kurt Hirschhorn, Professor of Pediatrics and Genetics, Chief, Division of Medical Genetics, Mount Sinai School of Medicine of The City University of New York; Dr. John W. Littlefield, Assistant Professor of Pediatrics at Harvard University, Department of Pediatrics, Massachusetts General Hospital, Boston; and, Dr. Arthur Robinson, Department of Pediatrics and Biophysiology, University of Colorado Medical Center. The first curriculum was planned in consultation with them, and reflected their experience and advice. The goal then was to train "assistants to physicians." Applicants were thought to need a "spread of mental capacities such as good retention, incisiveness, discipline, and ability to abstract logic." In addition, "any impression of intellectual ability, as well as motivation, are checked through a third procedure, namely, interviews. . . . by at least two persons." Beyond intellectual ability two major factors were carefully considered in accepting students—"pride tempered by humility and self confidence that a candidate can help fill this health need and has a determination to do so" (Richter 1968).

A grant from the Babcock Foundation supported the first year of the program. The curriculum for the opening year, 1969–1970, is listed in Table 1. The second year of the program included the content listed in Table 2. In 1970, and again in 1975, the Allied Health Manpower Training Division of the National Institutes of Health, awarded 5 year support to the program (DHEW Grant).

Eight students graduated from the program in 1971 (having pursued the above curriculum). Seven of these students were soon employed as genetic associates, the term then used for genetic counselors. Six began

Table 1. 1969–1970 Curriculum

Fall	Mendelian Molecular Genetics
	Probability and Elementary Statistics
	Human Genetics
Spring	Human Physiology
	Social Psychiatry
	Cytogenetics
	Medical Conferences at Mt. Sinai Hospital

Table 2. 1970–1971 Third and Fourth Semester Curriculum

Fall   Human Physiology
       Human Genetics
       Social Psychiatry

Spring   Laboratory Techniques—Cytogenetics
         Developmental Biology
         Clinic and Medical Conferences at Mt. Sinai and/or Einstein
         Clinics

---

work in New York City as counselors and one in Chicago. One enrolled in a doctoral program.

Development of an Interdisciplinary Curriculum

In the Fall of 1972 I joined the program as Co-Director. As a psychiatric social worker I had been exposed to families with children with developmental disabilities, but not specifically to patients with genetic diseases. I visited genetic centers in the New York area to see the manner in which diagnostic information was presented to families, and thus taught to the Sarah Lawrence students. I realized from those observations that the primary goal of counseling was the provision of medical information and genetic facts. Emotional responses to the diagnoses were studiously avoided. An atmosphere was created in which decision making was expected to be accomplished in a rational, logical way.

I felt the training of genetic counselors was seriously deficient without a major focus on counseling skills. I also thought that it was important to promote a psychosocial perspective in which patients would be viewed not as receptacles for genetic information, but as people in a crisis. That crisis involved not only receiving upsetting news but also the need to discuss painful subjects and/or to make difficult choices, frequently involving life or death issues. I was struck by the complexity of the problems families faced in coping with a genetic diagnosis. As we now recognize, the threat to one's self-esteem in such a crisis, as well as the resulting implications for marital stability, is often staggering. In 1972 these implications were rarely addressed and the toll of genetic diseases on individuals and society was sometimes barely recognized. A search for corroboration of my impressions revealed only a few references in the literature (Carter, Evans, Fraser-Roberts, and Buck, 1971; Leonard, Chase, and Childs 1972). However, in personal conversations with practicing geneticists there was considerable support for this perspective. Jessica

Davis, then co-director of the Sarah Lawrence program, was immediately supportive of changing the focus of the training to incorporate the psychological significance of being at risk for a genetic disease.

A major commitment was made in 1973 to expand the focus of the program. Then curricular decisions had to be made about introducing a body of knowledge that would promote the beginning counselors' awareness of psychological issues. If successful, this awareness would be deepened by exposure to actual patients in crisis. Although on-site supervision of trainees was then available, the medical model of information giving reigned. It remained the responsibility of the classroom to develop a comprehensive approach to patient care. This process involved first developing self-awareness skills, and then promoting the concept that patients/parents do not exist in a vacuum but are part of the larger family system (Minuchin and Fishman 1981). Even as late as 1981, Sorenson's study indicated that only 16% of the patients he studied had their sociomedical needs met in genetic counseling sessions (Sorenson, Swazey, and Scotch 1981).

Stephen Firestein, a psychotherapist, was recruited to develop the proposed curriculum. As I recall, Dr. Firestein observed only three genetic counseling sessions before consenting to the challenge presented to him. That was to create a curriculum for students to complement the rigorous science courses required to learn medical genetics. Unlike the course, Social Psychiatry, provided as an option to the first students in the program, Dr. Firestein's course, first offered in the Spring semester 1973, focused on psychodynamic concepts of personality development, including ego development, defense mechanisms, and family relationships. His course also required students to critique counseling sessions they observed. Students were to examine patients' needs and how the counseling met those needs, both verbal and unexpressed. Students found the course enlightening and in the 1973–1974 academic year it became, and remains, a two-semester course, Seminar in Genetic Counseling. In 1974 I began to meet with students to discuss their clinical experiences. It soon became clear that trainees needed to be taught basic counseling skills. Sheldon Reed was on the right track—a kind of genetic social worker could more effectively meet the informational needs of patients and families with hereditary problems! But providing information alone to families was no guarantee that clients would find it useful or even comprehend it. Counselors needed to learn how to structure a counseling session that would enable patients to "open up" to risk, revealing themselves as vulnerable or even unable to understand the genetics of their particular condition (Pellegrino and Thomasma 1988).

They would be able to do this only with counselors who had good therapeutic skills and who had enough self-confidence to handle the emotional material patients would reveal. A strong motivation to help would enable them to be objective even when patients made decisions contrary to the counselors best judgments. Out of these sessions with students a course entitled Issues in Genetic Counseling was developed. The course has evolved into a required three-semester sequence that conceptually bases genetic counseling on a psychosocial assessment of patients and/or families.

Another pivotal course introduced into the Sarah Lawrence counseling curriculum in 1976 is called Client Centered Counseling. This is an interview skills course based on Carl Rogers' concepts of nondirective counseling, employing empathic responses against the background of unconditional positive regard.

I would say that of all the counseling courses currently in our curriculum this course has had the greatest overall impact on our students. The course is taught in small groups in the first year of the program and essentially teaches students, for the first time, how to listen emphatically to another human being. The message is powerful and most students incorporate this approach in a fundamental way to their counseling perspective. Some students, however, have trouble integrating this perspective with the informational model to which they are eventually exposed and that they must incorporate into the overall genetic counseling model. It is my belief that the tension between these two communication models accounts for the confusion many genetic counselors experience with the issue of directiveness versus nondirectiveness. This

Table 3.   1991–1992 First Year Curriculum

Fall	Anatomy & Physiology
	Advanced Human Genetics
	Biochemistry Review (half semester)
	Cytogenetics/Biochemistry Lab
	Issues in Genetic Counseling I
	Client Centered Counseling
	Fieldwork
Spring	Anatomy & Physiology
	Biochemistry of Genetic Diseases
	Issues in Genetic Counseling I
	Client Centered Counseling
	Introduction to Clinical Medicine
	Delivery of Genetic Services
	Journal Club I
	Fieldwork

Table 4. 1991–1992 Second Year Curriculum

Fall	Medical Genetics
	Seminar in Genetic Counseling
	Issues in Genetic Counseling II
	Delivery of Genetic Services
	Journal Club II
	Thesis
	Clinical Rotations
Spring	Medical Genetics
	Seminar in Genetic Counseling
	Clinical Rotations
	AIDS Workshops (half semester)
	Thesis
	Orals

dilemma is eloquently discussed in the paper by Yarborough, Scott, and Dixon (1989).

At this time, students in the Sarah Lawrence program participate in four counseling courses: Issues in Genetic Counseling I and II, Client Centered Counseling, and Seminar In Genetic Counseling. They spend a total of 6 semesters developing the counseling skills I have just discussed.

In addition, other components of classes taught on a regular basis by practicing genetic counselors include the same emphasis in their teaching state-of-the-art genetic counseling. I think the Sarah Lawrence program is straightforward in offering interdisciplinary training in genetic counseling, with the balance tipping only slightly toward the sciences. I believe it is now valid to say that there **is** an established art and science of genetic counseling, however much it continues to evolve. Tables 3 and 4 lists the complete present Sarah Lawrence curriculum.

Masters Level Programs: Counseling Compoment

Twenty-one masters level programs are now training genetic counselors and 3 graduate nursing programs offer a specialization in genetic counseling. Many programs were established in consultation with existing programs; others have based their curricula on the recommendations documented, after a series of conferences, by Dumars et al. (1979) in "Genetic Associates: Their Training, Role, and Function," which recommended that programs include (1) Theory and Application of Interviewing and Counseling in Clinical Genetics and (2) Social, Ethical, and Legal Issues in Genetic Counseling. This report recommended didactic course work in two categories of a counseling nature.

Of the 21 counseling programs, 8 have a clearly defined counseling component with a philosophy of genetic counseling generally consistent with the focus previously described.

Genetic Counseling in the 1990s

The responsibilities the genetic counseling profession faces in educating the next generation of counselors are evolving quickly. They must be accompanied by thoughtful planning. There is a growing trend to train "single gene counselors," such as those who deal only with sickle cell counseling. This model may soon include cystic fibrosis counselors because of the crushing need for such health professionals now that the technology to test some cystic fibrosis carriers is available. The trend is likely to expand in light of the genetic markers for chronic diseases that human genome research will identify. I think it is important for the public to be protected from the development of health workers who are only partially trained and who assume, because of pressing sociomedical needs, responsibilities for guiding patients in areas where they have neither the basic knowledge nor the experience to counsel objectively or knowledgeably. Current safeguards operating in medical genetics and specifically developed to assure the integrity of the profession of medical genetics, namely American Board of Medical Genetics Certification of the genetic counseling team, should be rigorously maintained despite social pressures to lower standards of care. Why would one assume the families at risk for sickle cell disease, cystic fibrosis, or hypercholesterolemia deserve or require counseling that is likely to be less sensitive to the emotional, cultural, or informational needs of patients with rarer genetic diseases [such as any of the 5000 plus diseases catalogued by McKusick (1990)]. Sorenson effectively showed us at least 10 years ago that counselors who are not adept at dealing with most of the issues patients bring to a genetic counseling session are, in direct terms, inadequate.

It has been my intention in this chapter to focus on the importance of incorporating a psychodynamic approach to the care of patients at risk for genetic disease. Counselors whose training is abbreviated and whose skills are designed only to deal with one area of genetic risk will surely not have psychologically oriented training either. They will be deficient in all areas of counseling.

Now that the issues raised in genetic counseling are more complex, and the genetics more complicated, why would we settle for health practitioners less prepared to deal with these issues? Our commitment should be to train more people more adequately.

Value Neutrality in Genetic Counseling

The National Society of Genetic Counselors' (NSGC) Code of Ethics states that genetic counselors strive to

> enable their clients to make informed independent decisions, free of coercion, by providing or illuminating the necessary facts and clarifying the alternatives and anticipated consequences. (NSGC 1991a)

Two verbs are significant here—*illuminating* necessary facts and *clarifying* alternatives. This proactive description of the genetic counselor signifies not only the responsibility the counselor has to assist in patient decision making, but implies that the counselor's role in patient decision making is integral to the responsible discharge of his/her duties. Kessler (1980) writes persuasively that "the genetic counselor's interventions, or lack thereof, may have major long-term consequences for the counselees." These descriptions seem far afield from the person-centered counseling of Carl Rogers, in which empathic responses and unconditional positive regard are designed to enable patients to become fully functioning individuals, able to make appropriate, constructive decisions on their own.

The ethos of genetic counseling suggests that genetic counselors can be effective only by maintaining an objective, nondirective stance. It seems more realistic and more constructive to teach genetic counseling trainees that their personal values and opinions will probably influence their counseling, unless they are unusually diligent in recognizing their biases.

Once they have identified their biases, which can range from religious attitudes to a dislike for people whose physical characteristics they find distasteful, the belief is that they can control their influence in the genetic counseling encounter. There is little evidence to support this belief. During many years of interviewing applicants to graduate school, only twice have I heard a student state that personal religious views about abortion might interfere with the ability to counsel patients objectively. In contrast, the 1988 Eighth Annual Educational Conference of the National Society of Genetic Counselors included a workshop on "The Genetic Counselor With a Strong Religious Or Spiritual Identity." During this workshop several experienced counselors spoke about the pain they felt in discussing pregnancy terminations with patients. Some counselors even talked about sleep disturbances they suffered when their counselees made decisions to terminate a pregnancy due to genetic reasons.

There is no known way to completely block the influence of one's personal views on the issues genetic counselors discuss with patients, and few counselors are adept at identifying the extent to which their views influence the counseling. Thus it seems incumbent on training programs to provide considerable opportunity during the 2 years of training to examine this issue and to enable students to recognize the origin and development of their personal values and attitudes. As counselors encourage patients to "open up" in counseling sessions, so must counselors "open up to themselves" in their training. This process can be difficult for students and counseling therapy is often a recommended means of assisting the process.

Conclusion

Our society is not one that has easily adapted to the concept that we can and must make choices regarding health-related issues. While there have been no careful analytic studies it is my impression that such choices are particularly difficult when they involve issues related to the quality of life of our progeny. We must anticipate and therefore prepare our students to deal with a whole range of issues involving genetic risk. As we become better able to identify and quantify such risks, owing in part to the advances of the genome project, it is incumbent on those of us responsible for the training of genetic counselors to continually adapt to the new opportunities that research opens up. It will be particularly challenging to provide counseling without value judgment. It is important to recognize that we cannot as genetic counselors alter risk or be perceived as able to provide a means for risk avoidance; rather, we can provide counseling as effectively as our present knowledge and technology permit to help cope with the potential consequences of known genetic risk. This includes risk that relates to the individual, as is the case when we are able to identify the genetic markers that place a person at risk for smoking-related lung cancer, for example, as well as the identification of genetic markers that would place potential progeny at risk for cystic fibrosis. These new dimensions of genetic counseling will obligate the counselor to become even more involved in deeper levels of counselee decision making than current practice requires.

We run many risks as we go forward with adapting our training programs for genetic counselors to the rapidly advancing knowledge of the human genome. It is likely that the greatest risk would result from not assuming responsibility for training people in state-of-the-art genetic science and in placing this training in the appropriate psychosocial context.

Chapter 3

The Workplace Ideology of Genetic Counselors

CHARLES BOSK

Introduction

The purpose of this chapter is to assess the status of a nondirective ethos in genetic counseling today. I will carry out this assessment by concentrating on the following four questions:

1. What is a nondirective ethos?
2. Are the nondirective ethos and value neutrality different concepts? If so, how do they differ?
3. What are the behaviors of genetic counselors and their clients in the clinical setting?
4. What are the ways in which value neutrality and nondirective counseling are and are not implemented in practice?

Before proceeding it is necessary to make a number of disclaimers. First, I will be answering all these questions under conditions of extreme uncertainty. I am an ethnographer; the description asked for in questions three and four will be full of everyday detail, a rich report of one "shop floor culture" of genetic counselors, the team at Nightingale Children's Center (a pseudonym), whom I followed around (for such are ethnographic methods) at the turn of the last decade (Bosk 1992).

My analytic task, which was not entirely self-imposed, was to describe the counselor–client relationship as it was understood in the context of the genetic counseling service of an elite, urban pediatric center. My purpose was to show how a group of professionals defined their mission, performed their core task, and understood their shared identity and fate (Bucher and Strauss 1961).

I can describe in great specificity the behaviors of counselors and clients in one place at one point in time as "exemplars" of "value-neutrality" (Kuhn 1977). It was hard to assess at the time how representative the exemplars were, the everyday routines, and session strategies that the counselors likened to "songs and dance," which I observed. Did their collective and individual acting out in a self-conscious way a "nondirective ethos" and "value neutrality" mirror all genetic counselors? Were they a good group from which to discover a set of behavioral markers? Further, it is hard now for me to assess how all the changes in the world, in health care, and in genetics of the last 10 years have changed interpretations of "nondirective/value-neutral" work ethic of genetic counselors, although that they have done so seems unarguable.

Three changes are so basic as to demand comment. First, at the time of my fieldwork, ethical concerns were an unpredictable occurrence with only inchoate workplace routines for resolving serious problems. Since I made my observations these concerns have become routinized and bureaucratized in the institutional structure of the contemporary tertiary care center. Institutional Review Boards (IRBs), ethics committees, and clinical bioethicists are now familiar actors with definite roles to play in care. The genetic counselors whom I will discuss were much more alone with their uncertainties and doubts than need be the case today. How effectively these new "support" structures work is, of course, a question about which precious little is known. Nonetheless, the very fact that institutionalized channels exist for routing such questions surely has some impact on those working on clinical frontiers, which are problematic. At the very least, an institutional mechanism now exists for dealing with "troubles" in the definition of proper action or for approving breaches of "nondirective/value-neutral" action to serve some other goal.

Second, much of the work of genetic counseling that was a jealously guarded prerogative of the physicians of Nightingale Children's Center has now become a standard part of obstetrical care. Consequently, much of the work that at Nightingale was done only by genetic counselors is now done by nurses, social workers, or Master's level genetic counselors as part of ambulatory care in the community. How deeply these workers internalized a spirit of "nondirective/value-neutrality" is one question and how they use it is another.

This alerts us to something that we need to pay close attention to—the services that are thought of as genetic counseling are dispensed by many who would not claim the title. Conversely, as therapeutic applications become available, the attachments of the geneticists who develop them to "nondirective/value-neutrality" is likely to be weaker than that of the everyday genetic counselors. It is a mistake to expect these research entrepreneurs to be "value-neutral" and "nondirective" when discussing their innovations. The culture of clinical research is a very different occupational culture than the one I am about to describe (Fox 1959; Fox and Swazey 1974). Nonetheless, we may expect enthusiasm to be constrained by the institutional developments described—the complex bureaucratic structure that decides ethical questions for the hospital involved.

Third, we have become increasingly aware of some of the ambiguities of health care. Not quite a firmly entrenched right and something more than an ordinary consumer good, we do not collectively have a good grip on health care. All that we know for certain is that health care is a scarce good, that its allocation and distribution are problematic, and paradoxical. Those in intensive care units who may want less health care have as much trouble having their expectations met as those who are uninsured and want more.

When thinking about clinical implications of advances in genetics, there is a tendency to be dazzled by the rather spectacular cosmological, metaphysical dilemmas that are posed and to miss altogether the prosaic collective, distributional questions. Even so, at an every day level, like all health care workers, genetic counselors are asked to be managers and conservers of scarce resources. This, too, may exert an impact on the operation of an ideology of "nondirectiveness/value-neutrality."

The Workplace Ideology of Genetic Counseling

A workplace ideology is a set of values, working rules of thumb, and self-evident truth shared by workers about everyday problems, proper solutions, or acceptable explanations when things go awry. A nondirective ethos is one of the two main elements in the workplace ideology of the genetic counselor; the other is a principled stance of value-neutrality. Both serve to limit the role of genetic counselor to "information-giver" (Hsia 1979) or "decision-facilitator" (Antley 1979).

Such limitation is important for keeping decisions based on genetic information private. Genetic counselors seek to accomplish a number of goals. First, they seek to distance themselves from earlier, state-imposed practices of genetics. "Nondirectiveness" serves to ensure that client decisions are voluntary and uncoerced unlike the involuntary, coercive State Eugenics of earlier eras (Hubbard 1986; Müller-Hill 1988; Haller 1963; Ludmerer 1972).

In practice, "nondirectiveness" means a reluctance to make therapeutic recommendations. This reluctance derives from the fact that often the only option available is second-trimester abortion. "Nondirectiveness" then serves to help genetic counselors to avoid the pariah status that Imber (1986) finds clings to physicians who perform abortions. At the same time it allows counselors to avoid confronting any unexpected moral parallels and problems with the practice of eugenics. By confirming genetic counseling practice to private pay settings where decisions are clearly voluntary, counselors can avoid claims of coerced reproductive decisions.

To think of nondirectiveness pragmatically and situationally, imagine yourself observing a genetic counseling session. A bottom line risk figure has been given to a couple for a nondiagnosable, *in utero* recessive disorder. The husband or wife turns to the genetic counselor and asks, "What would you do?" A paragon of nondirectiveness might answer "What I would do is unimportant. What is important is that you as a couple make a decision that is consistent with your own beliefs and values." A persistent couple might continue the questioning, "What do others in our situation do?"

This second question presents a conflict between the nondirectiveness of the genetic counselor and his/her tasks as an information giver and decision-facilitator. For this information will be used to guide choice—by providing it the counselor will have been directive. The counselors I observed generally declined to comment on the "typical decision of others" when asked to do so by couples. Rather, they used the occasion of the questions to refocus the discussion to the couple's individual decision. Occasionally, couples who were unusually curious about "those in our position" were referred to self-help and support groups if their particular disease had one.

Value-neutrality is, along with nondirectiveness, an element of workplace ideology designed to assure that genetic knowledge will not be abused in its applications. Value-neutrality is of a piece with other values in medical culture in a way that nondirectiveness is not. (In most domains of medicine, a sustained instrumental activism on the clients' behalf replaces nondirectiveness.) Value-neutral medical professionals do not judge their clients and their choices. The goal of counseling is not to get clients to enact the counselors' values, but rather to get the clients to realize their own. As elements of workplace ideology, both nondirectiveness and value-neutrality shift the focus of counseling from outcomes to the process by which outcomes are achieved. Both values are said to serve patient autonomy but they may equally well, depending on the occasion, serve to limit counselors' emotional involvement by restricting expertise to facts neutrally conveyed.

Although a nondirective style and value-neutrality are the dominant ideology under which genetic counselors practice, they are not the only ones. Kessler (1980) noted a paradigm shift in counseling with greater concern being paid to psychological issues. Twiss (1979) has called for counselors to acknowledge the ways in which they act as moral advisors. Such acknowledgment calls for abandonment of both value-neutrality and a nondirective style as the issue warrants. Yarborough, Scott, and Dixon (1989) show how a commitment to a nondirective style can thwart the goal of patient autonomy that it is intended to foster. In addition, the work of Wertz and Fletcher (1988) indicates great cross-national variation in the workplace ideology of genetic counselors. The same survey work indicates that there also is great individual variation in counselor response to specific problems. While a nondirective/value-neutral style may be the normative ideal, it is apparent that is not always achieved.

Moreover, clearly value-neutrality and nondirectiveness themselves were adopted to the degree they were because of the absence of any treatment for genetic ills save therapeutic abortions. As treatments develop, it makes sense to expect that value-neutrality and nondirection may disappear as workplace values. Health care is not full of scientific entrepreneurs chary of offering the benefits of the therapies that they have developed. Traditionally with innovations the pattern is one of over-enthusiasm, extensive early use, and then finally more limited application as the pitfalls and promises of innovation become better understood. Moreover, as counseling spreads down the medical hierarchy and out of the hospital, the gulf between those providing counseling and those doing innovative research will grow. There is little reason to suspect that those who develop new therapies will share the appreciation of value-neutrality and a nondirective style that characterizes current genetic counselors. But perhaps this assessment underestimates the commitments of the genetic counseling community. Anyway, the time has come to describe the recent past rather than speculate about the near future.

What Counselors Do

As medical professionals, genetic counselors are a sociological paradox: they are professionals whose knowledge base is as complex and as abstract as any imaginable, yet they—by choice—exert virtually no power—nor constrain any autonomy of their clients. Those I observed were information specialists, neutral staters of odds, problem experts, and decision facilitators rather than decision makers. They perform socially enabling work either for their lay clients or for other physicians who consult them at Nightingale Children's Center.

With lay clients counseling practices are remarkably stereotyped. Counseling is usually completed in a single session. The content of the session is summarized in a postclinic follow-up letter. Counselors are concerned about "the story" they tell to clients. Good stories contain clear diagnostic labels, precise recurrence risks, and the possibility of prenatal diagnosis. Bad stories are full of uncertainty—the diagnosis or the mode of inheritance is uncertain, or the prenatal diagnosis is tricky. Counselors generally prefer good stories to bad ones (clients with bad stories are said to be suffering from "the vagues").

However, counselors tell good stories and bad stories in the same way. First, in nondirective fashion, they ask their clients what questions they want answered; they elicit the clients' agenda. But, most commonly, this elicitation is bare politeness, it plays little role in how the genetic counselor proceeds. Counseling is the passing of technical information to clients; the emphasis on the counselors' part is on the quality of the information transmitted and not on how it is understood or acted on.

There are a number of ritual features of that transmission that are noteworthy. First, scientific thoroughness and technical proficiency are marked in a number of ways. The weekly preclinic conference discussion of what to tell parents centers not on who the parents are, what their level of understanding is, or what the amount of their distress is, but instead on what the literature says about the genetic condition in question. It is as if each genetic condition has its own "complete story" that needs to be told independent of the clients being counseled.

For the most exotic condition, counselors initiate phone contacts with "big names" at other institutions to make certain that no recent developments that have implications for *in utero* diagnosis have escaped their attention. A number of encyclopedias of birth anomalies are kept on hand during clinic, so findings from clinical exams can be correlated with available data. The emphasis is quite clearly on genetics as a science rather than counseling as a relational process.

During sessions with parents, counselors use a number of devices to dramatize that either they have an explanation for a child's aberrant development or that they can assign a specific risk to a pregnancy. When a problem was chromosomal, the counselors always displayed the photographic karyotype, a picture of chromosomes taken through a microscope;

Bill Smith (a pseudonym for a genetic counselor at Nightingale Children's Center) is meeting with the Chilmarks, a couple whose child is in the neonatal intensive care unit. Bill begins the discussion: "I think we have as much of an answer as we are ever going to get. Your baby has an extra piece of chromosomal material. Look at the karyotype we did of your baby [here he passes the picture to the parents]. The 21 is here, part of it seems to be missing but it's really here at the bottom of this chromosome [he points to

13]. On banding, we see that most of the 21 is here. The top is equivalent to 13, but 13 is trisomic, that means there are three pieces of it.

This routine display of photographs and the expert decoding of them is a regular feature of counseling for couples who come in for advanced maternal age (women over 35 years old are by far the largest single segment of clients who used counseling services). Ultrasound photographs and karyotypes are shown to parents to help aid their understanding of how prenatal diagnosis works. They are evidence of the real problem.

Of course, such photographic displays can only be a feature of chromosomal disorders. Other types of disorders call for different dramatizations of scientific expertise. For recessive disorders, counselors draw Mendelian diagrams for prospective parents to enable them to understand their reproductive risks better. There are cases when counselors cannot display the problem in a photography or display recurrence risks in a diagram. On these occasions, counselors deliver long didactic lectures on specific genetic disorders.

> Albert Samuels (also a pseudonym) is counseling the Menemshas, a couple who has a child with an antibody deficiency. He begins the session: 'What I have to tell you today is very complicated—there's no clear answer why Teddy has his antibody deficiency. You're going to have to know an awful lot about genetics to follow what I say. We have to assume it's a genetic problem. Now there are many problems with antibody deficiencies that are inherited. . . . Now, let's start at the beginning. Genes come in pairs, and there are thousands of them on chromosomes. Now when sperm fertilizes an egg, each takes on a chromosome, so there's a 50–50 chance of any member of a gene pair being inherited from a mother or a father. Now in these antibody disorders, there are three modes of inheritance. They can either be sex-linked, recessive, or a new mutation. . . ' Samuels then goes on to explain each of these and their associated recurrence risk.

The counselors' explanation of genetic diseases explained cause to parents in impersonal, distant, abstract, technical terms: "This part of the photograph where the arrow is" or "we all have bad genes. It's just an anomoly, a random and tragic accident that these genes get passed on in just the right order to produce conditions like Kevin has." To soften the blow in having a child born with birth defects, the genetic counselor speaks of normal birth as a "symphonic" miracle. Yet, in translating their understanding of why this miracle fails to occur, the genetic counselors are forced into an everyday language that makes this miracle a mundane matter of proper switching and correct copying. Problems of neural tube development, for example, are always analogized to zippers functioning properly. To demonstrate neural tube development, genetic counselors always fold paper into tubes.

Their relentless focus on the scientific and technical side of client troubles permits counselors to dramatize their expertise and to avoid engaging the raft to emotional issues raised by the presence of genetic disease. In fact, the genetic counselors often find managing this emotional work outside the specific domain of their expertise. So much is this the case that this work is routinely "turfed" to the genetic associate, who despite the general prohibition against them seeing patients is allowed to meet with them for this "nonspecialized" part of the counseling tasks.

> I remember feeling somewhat confused the first time that Bill said to me, "go in and mop-up." I mean I just didn't know what that meant when I first started here. I have since learned that what it means is to just sit and let people talk. But they do not want to do that with another person.

Not only was the genetic associate used in this way, but I was often assigned to observe those cases that the genetic counselors assumed would have the heaviest emotional overtones. Often I was asked to interview these patients following their sessions. As a researcher, I was thus coopted into providing "mop-up" services as well.

It is not that the genetic counselors are unaware of the emotional wear and tear of genetic problems. They are. It is not that counselors are unaware of how difficult reproductive decision making can be. They are. Bill, for example, said he knew when there were emotional troubles in a session because he "gets a headache." Counselors routinely encourage couples to talk about these troubles, but not with them. When a couple mentioned emotional difficulties in coping the genetic counselors responded with the ritualistic injunction, "talking helps." The category of people with whom "talking" might be helpful included family, "people who have gone through something similar" (especially those connected to organized support groups, friends, clergy, and mental health professions). During the time of my research, the genetic counseling unit at Nightingale never established an effective liaison with psychiatric or social services. Finally, it is interesting to note that the genetic counselor never included themselves in the list of people with whom talk is helpful. Emotional troubles are a personal issue, a family issue, a communal issue, or an issue for the professionals; they are not a question properly addressed in the professional relationship of counselor and client. Rather, counselors use such questions to highlight a couple's autonomy and privacy as they point them toward other resources.

As they go about their work, a constant refrain of the genetic counselors is that the standard for good work is not a couple's decision but the information the counselor provides for making that decision. Counselors remind each other that "they do not hand out genes nor plan pregnancies." When pressed by patients for recommendations, the genetic counselors, as noted above, refuse to give them.

> At the postclinic conference, Berger (yet another pseudonym) reported on seeing the parents of a child who had just been born with an open myelomeningecele. The parents had decided to place the child in a residential home and not to repair the neural-tube defect. Berger reported that he had done "standard" myelo counseling.
>
> The couple, continued Berger, was "comfortable" with the decision not to treat and were "leery" of today's session because somewhere along the line "they had been exposed to someone who had challenged the decision, perhaps a sister-in-law."
>
> Berger said it was not the task of the center to have them do so. 'Our job here is not to convince parents to do one thing or another. We provide information. We make sure that they are comfortable with what it is that they are going to do.'"

Berger's explicit announcement of the group's mission is noteworthy since he is its most senior member and its formal leader. Also, it presents a paradox: How, if the parents did not want to discuss the decision, could Berger evaluate if they were comfortable with it? In fact, does not the parent's insistence on keeping this particular Pandora's Box closed speak to a certain level of discomfort? However, such discomfort is emotional and hence outside the mandate of the Center and its workers. There is an interactional contradiction that inheres in the practice of genetic counseling at Nightingale Children's Center. A commitment to nondirection requires a certain reticence to explore issues couples would prefer to keep closed. Yet a commitment to decisions "couples are comfortable with" requires a certain amount of unpleasant prying.

Breaches of Shop Floor Ideology

Counselors attempted to avoid the most problematic aspect of their task by confining themselves to scientific information and impersonal risk statements. Such a task definition they felt was the only way to allow patients to make their own decisions—it was the only way to preserve a couples' autonomy in the private business of reproductive decision making. Nonetheless counselors often delivered risk statements in a manner that undercut their formal commitment to nondirective counseling.

For example, the bulk of the patients offered prenatal diagnosis had as their presenting problem "advanced maternal age." In these cases, the genetic counselors spoke of amniocentesis as a device for reducing parental anxiety and providing reassurance:

Giordano (yes, another pseudonym) is counseling a couple who has recently lost a child in a drowning accident. The mother is forty, she feels "funny" about wanting another child. She wonders if she is "too old to be a mother." Giordano begins to explain amniocentesis. The chances overall are 2–3% of having a kid with a birth defect. But, the chance of Downs syndrome increases with age. Look [Giordano takes a piece of paper and draws a graph], if this is the age of mothers and this is the chance of having a kid with Downs, you can see the following: For a twenty year old, the chance of having a baby with Downs is one in 1500 and it stays like that till about age 29 when it begins to climb. It gradually climbs until about 35. Then it really goes up, so that the chances among 35 and 40 of having a child with Downs syndrome are between one in 250. With this test, we can bring your odds back to those of a twenty year old.

When discussing amniocentesis, counselors often claimed the procedure brought the risk of having an affected child down to "below" the normal population risks since many risks for the population were screened for by the procedure.

In general, when a prenatal screening mechanism existed for a condition, it was offered to parents with the same enthusiasm that amniocentesis was offered to women of advanced maternal age. Couples were reassured their chances of having a perfect baby were higher than average. Genetic counselors neutralized whatever stigma adhered to their work as "abortion counselors" by reminding themselves and others that first, a significant number of couples who would not have borne children but for the services that the counseling center was able to provide, did so; and second, patients were never coerced, they remained free to make their own choices.

In addition, counselors routinely breach their nondirective/value-neutral ethos because of the way that they shape factual information to couples. The crux here is understanding the construction of risk statements. First, all risk statements are comparative. One goal of counseling is to have prospective parents understand their own risks in relation to the normal population risk. The normal population risk that counselors quote to their clients is 3%. This is a figure that surprises most clients who assume that birth is less risky than that.

On the one hand, the very fact that risks can be expressed in numeric form allows counselors, if they choose, to merely pass on information to clients in an objective fashion; i.e., "the normal population risk is 3%, your risk is 6%." Such precise statements underscore the counselor's objectivity, neutrality, and commitment to scientific data. However, such risk statements without elaboration are rare. On the other hand, the numeric form of risk statements allows counselors to inform couples in ways that imply what a reasonable and responsible person will do with the information. For example, consider the difference between the following statements, each of which is correct: "your risk is 3% greater than the general population," and "your risk is double the general population." Risk statements are more than bare unelaborated numbers despite the counselors commitment to not intruding on private decision making. Counselors framed risk statements so that couples could either appreciate the seriousness or the triviality of a problem.

These two deviations notwithstanding, the counselor's dedication to a nondirective/value-neutral ethos is heroic. On those rare occasions when this ethos was violated by one of the group the others were visibly distressed. All violations were seen as intrusive and unwarranted; all were to be avoided. Counselors adopted a nondirective/value-neutral ethos not only when counseling lay couples but also when answering the questions of their colleagues at Nightingale who asked them to consult. Most frequently these consultations involve neonatologists who are unsure whether or not to treat severely compromised neonates.

The neonatologists at Nightingale well understand that not initiating treatment is easier than discontinuing it once it has begun. Even so, not initiating treatment is a very difficult decision. This decision is made easier for them if a lethal genetic abnormality that would make treatment futile is discovered. If such is the case neonatologists feel a decision not to treat is morally justified. Without such a finding, this decision is more difficult.

> Bill Smith and Al Samuels have been called to the neonatal intensive care unit. The neonatologist wants to do a bone-marrow tap rather than a standard venipuncture to find out as soon as possible if a child has trisomy 18.
>
> Both of them examine the baby. They agree that it is a "bad" baby with problems. However, neither think that those problems are chromosomal. Both agree a bone marrow is not necessary.
>
> Bill reports this to the baby's attending physician. He asks Bill if it is possible to rule trisomy 18 out completely without a karyotype. He says it is not. The attending says he is uncomfortable with a child on a ventilator as long as trisomy 18 is a possibility. He wants the marrow for karyotyping, does Bill agree that it is "necessary" for the quickest diagnosis. He does. The attending calls hematology.
>
> Samuels, Bill and I retreat to a side room. Samuels begins to complain, "This is ridiculous. Everybody can see this is a bad baby. . . ." Samuels keeps up his litany of complaint about misallocated resources, unnecessary procedures, and treating attending anxiety rather than taking care of patients.
>
> At this last comment Bill grows testy and barks back at Samuels: "Enough already. I know you think it's a bad baby. I think it's a bad baby, too. But, that is not the point. It's not the question. Look, you want to put on a green

scrub suit and take care of these patients, fine. Then you can decide what tests need to be done or not. I am a consultant. He told me he would be helped by the test, and I ordered it for him. I said okay."

Samuels said it was a matter of judgment and that he disagreed with the attending in this case.

Bill agreed: "Yes it is a matter of judgment—and if you want to make the final judgment, then you have to take care of the patients. Otherwise, it's my job as a consultant to help attendings in whatever way they ask for."

Samuels, it is worth noting, disagreed with the handling of this case and not with the definition of consultant responsibility.

So, a nondirective value-neutral ethos marks the relations of counselors with colleagues every bit as much as it does their relations with clients. This is so even though his/her stance may serve to undermine the client autonomy that the ethos is said to protect. Although formally equal, the genetic counselors never exercise any of those prerogatives one might expect when colleagues disagree. They do not push their own point of view. They do not even use the device of the gentle question to get their colleagues to reconsider courses of action that they consider ill advised. For them, "consultant ethos" means providing their colleagues what they want, even when they know that this runs counter to parental wishes.

Nonetheless, the counselors do worry about families whom they feel are trapped by their overzealous colleagues. Yet despite their obvious concern, all the genetic counselors do is wring their hands and trade their anxieties in private. They neither ally themselves with parents nor inform colleagues of their worries. They are a virtual Greek Chorus commenting on a tragedy that they are well placed to observe but powerless to prevent.

Conclusion

In the early years of the 1980s the genetic counselors (all of whom were physicians) I observed used a value-neutral/nondirective ideology to preserve patient autonomy. Very often, having emotional needs addressed was the price that users of the service paid for their autonomy. It is hard to assess how the changes of the last decade have affected the work of genetic counselors. It may be that the new generation of genetic counselors trained in master's programs found a way to cleave to the workplace ideology of their predecessors at the same time that they more clearly meet clients emotional needs. It may be that their good intentions are stymied by organizational arrangements. In any case, these new workers deserve the same amount of attention that researchers have given genetic counselors who are M.D.s or Ph.D.s.

In addition, as knowledge expands, and especially as treatments develop, the nondirective/value-neutral ideology will come under intense pressure. For once something beneficial can be offered, health care workers have generally had trouble not being enthusiastic about offering it. It will be interesting to see how the tension between "doing good" and "preserving autonomy" works itself out in the field of genetic counseling.

Chapter 4

When Theory Meets Practice: Challenges to the Field of Genetic Counseling

BONNIE S. LEROY

The Human Genome Project is a major international undertaking utilizing the expertise of many scientific disciplines. The hope is that information gained through this project will aid in research. Genetic research may provide clues to questions such as, how do cells become different from one another in early embryonic life? What controls cell aging and reproduction? and Just how do humans fit in the evolutionary ladder? Answers to these questions and others will help us better understand ourselves and our relationships to other life with which we share the earth. Hopefully they will also provide answers about the origin of common diseases such as cancer and mental illness.

The promises of the Human Genome Project provoke thought about ethical issues in genetic counseling now and in the future. This chapter will describe genetic risks, review the basic tenets of genetic counseling, and evaluate our struggle with ethical issues faced in assembling a presymptomatic testing program for Huntington disease. Finally, a case study will illustrate some ethical conflicts and policy challenges.

How Are Genetic Conditions Transmitted?

All of us carry recessive genes that are capable of resulting in a birth defect or disorder in our offspring. In most cases individuals are fortunate enough to have children with a partner whose abnormal recessive genes are different from their own. However, some people are not so fortunate.

Thousands of children are born each year with a genetic birth defect or disorder because their parents are both carriers of a recessive disease. Because it is not yet possible to screen for the presence of all known gene abnormalities, a couple usually first discovers they are both carriers of a genetic condition when they have an affected child. The possibility of population "gene screening" may be in our future.

Most of us also carry genes that play a role in the development of common adult conditions such as cancer, diabetes, and heart disease. Presently, we use known risk factors such as family history and life-style to predict who may be at a high risk. Empiric data on affected individuals and their families aid in risk assessment for these conditions. Some individuals go through early adult life waiting to see if they have escaped the "family disease." With new information gained through the Human Genome Project, it may be possible to identify high-risk individuals with gene testing.

Many genetic conditions are inherited in a dominant fashion placing the offspring of an affected parent at a 50% risk of also being affected. Most of these conditions do not affect health until later in life, which means that children of an affected parent will not know if they too must deal with the effects of the disease until symptoms appear or until they have outlived their statistical risk. However, presymptomatic testing for a few of these conditions is already available.

Because anyone of reproductive age is capable of having a child with a genetic disorder and most of us carry genetic risk factors for common adult conditions, we are all potential genetic counseling patients and will likely be affected by the knowledge gained through the Human Genome Project.

The Basic Tenets of Genetic Counseling

Dr. Sheldon Reed, Professor Emeritus at the University of Minnesota, coined the term "genetic counseling" in 1947. In his book, he describes genetic counseling as being "a most important practical application of the findings of the science of human genetics. It could help almost every family, if available to them." In his chapter on "A Philosophy for Counseling," he discusses dealing with patients at their own level, providing people with an understanding of their genetic problems and providing individuals with their reproductive options so that they can make the decision that is best for them (Reed 1980).

The elements of genetic counseling were defined (American Society of

Human Genetics 1975) in a 1975 report to the American Society of Human Genetics by an Ad Hoc Committee on Genetic Counseling. This report discusses genetic counseling as "a communication process which deals with the human problems associated with the occurrence, or the risk of occurrence, of a genetic disorder in a family." The report elaborates on the process that involves communicating facts to families in a way they can understand so that they can choose a course of action appropriate for them. In 1991, the National Society of Genetic Counselors adopted a Professional Code of Ethics. The section, "Genetic Counselors and Their Clients," includes a discussion of respect for clients' beliefs, background and culture, and the counselor's duty to enable clients to make autonomous decisions by providing all necessary information (National Society of Genetic Counselors 1991). All professionals educated to provide genetic counseling are taught that genetic counseling should be

1. Educational
2. Nondirective
3. Unconditional
4. Supportive

Genetic counselors strive to educate patients and families about genetic condition(s) in a nondirective fashion. The goal is to allow individuals to make choices based on their personal backgrounds and beliefs and not those of the counselor. Genetic counselors also strive to provide support on an unconditional basis. Individuals may choose to have testing or not, and choose how to use the results of the testing or the information in the counseling session as they see best. We value patient autonomy. These are the basics of genetic counseling. This is what I was taught more than 10 years ago and this is what I now teach as director of a graduate program in genetic counseling.

These genetic counseling values have served me well in my practice. An ethical issue would pop up now and then, such as a discovering of false paternity, or a request for prenatal testing so a couple could select the gender of their next child. Fortunately, there always seemed to be either a set precedent or an institutional policy dictating how one should deal with these issues and others.

Three years ago the University of Minnesota began offering presymptomatic testing for Huntington disease. I have found this type of testing to be riddled with ethical issues for which there are no precedents and which sometimes challenge the established foundations of genetic counseling. Evaluating our experiences can serve as a prototype for other testing options that may become available in the future through the information gained from the Human Genome Project.

A Presymptomatic Testing Program for Huntington disease

Huntington Disease is a genetic disorder inherited in an autosomal dominant fashion. Offspring of an affected parent have a 50% risk of inheriting the gene. To our knowledge, all who inherit the gene develop the disorder; however, the age of onset varies in individuals within and between families. Most people exhibit symptoms between 35 and 45 years of age, although some show symptoms before age 20 and others do not develop manifestations of the disease until age 65 or greater. Huntington disease is a progressive neurodegenerative disorder resulting in uncontrolled movements, dementia, and psychiatric symptoms. The course of the disease is usually 15 to 20 years from onset of symptoms. At this time, there is no effective therapy to cure or slow the progression of the condition. The primary genetic defect causing Huntington disease remains unknown.

In 1983, James Gusella et al. published their work describing a genetic marker linked to the Huntington disease gene (Gusella et al. 1983). This marker is a normal variation in human DNA. That is to say, there are normal differences in our genetic information that do not cause problems but are useful in that they allow scientists to tell us apart on the genetic level. This marker allowed geneticists, for the first time, to follow the Huntington disease gene through many families predicting which individuals were at a very high risk for developing the disease. Since 1983 many new markers linked to the gene have been discovered and increasingly accurate testing is an option for affected families. As one can imagine, we have encountered many ethical issues with this test. For the first time, at-risk individuals need to decide if they really want to know whether they will develop a deteriorating disease. Insurance companies may want this information before issuing life insurance to an at-risk individual. Employers may want to know if an employee will develop a condition that could affect judgment and place the employee and perhaps the public at risk for accidents.

In 1988, the presymptomatic testing program at the University of Minnesota was developed by Dr. Leonard Heston, a psychiatrist with research interests in Alzheimer disease and the affective disorders. Dr. Heston saw this testing as a prototype for similar testing for Alzheimer disease and some psychiatric illnesses when genetic markers become available. The molecular diagnostics laboratory, directed by Dr. Harry Orr, obtained the DNA markers needed for testing.

The testing protocol we developed is service, rather than research oriented with no grant money available to help patients with expenses. Patients utilize their health insurance for payment or pay out of pocket. Many individuals choose to pay out of pocket for fear that their health insurance will be canceled should the test results show that they most likely have the gene. Some patients are also concerned more generally about confidentiality.

Since we set no residency requirements, patients from outside Minnesota wishing testing initially needed to travel to the University of Minnesota multiple times to complete the protocol. In 1991 we expanded the laboratory services to accept specimens from other testing centers. Samples are accepted only from centers able to provide genetic counseling services, neurologic and neuropsychometric evaluation services, and supportive counseling services. Individuals interested in presymptomatic testing for Huntington disease must follow a set protocol for evaluation and counseling. At risk individuals must have a documented positive family history for Huntington disease and must provide records confirming the diagnosis in the family, or go through a diagnostic workup at the University of Minnesota before tests will be done. No results will be given over the phone, only in person. Follow-up counseling is required. All patients are strongly encouraged to include a companion (spouse, friend, parent, counselor) during their testing process, which proceeds as follows:

Visit 1   Intake counseling, family history, medical history, genetic counseling, confirmation of diagnosis of affected family members with review of records or exam, and psychological evaluation.

Visit 2   Neurologic evaluation and psychometric testing. Review of genetics and psychological counseling.

Visit 3   Second psychological evaluation and counseling, blood collection from proband and consent forms signed.

Visit 4   Discussion of results.

Visit 5   Follow-up counseling

The protocol was designed to offer presymptomatic testing to at-risk individuals and at the same time to provide psychological support throughout the testing process. Multiple visits are required to allow time to decide not to have the testing, to postpone the results, or to feel comfortable about their decision to complete the testing process. Multiple visits also allow us to feel we are obtaining truly informed consent and that we are preparing the patient as much as possible for any adverse outcomes. Individuals excluded from testing include the following:

1.   Patients found to be symptomatic on examination.
2.   Patients with an existing psychiatric illness or with a history of a suicide attempt.
3.   Patients under 18 years of age.

4. Patients being asked to have testing by a second party. (e.g., another family member, insurance company, employer, etc.).

The testing procedure usually follows an initial telephone intake where the caller, not always the patient, is provided information about the protocol and costs. The telephone intake is also the time when the family history is evaluated for the possibility of successful laboratory testing. Many families cannot be tested as the individuals necessary for the analysis are either not available or will not provide blood samples. If a family can be evaluated from a laboratory standpoint, written information is mailed to the family about the protocol and costs. It is the responsibility of the patient to contact the family members who need to provide blood samples for testing. In most families, six to eight members are needed for accurate linkage testing. The genetic counselor is available to answer questions from any family member but the request to participate must come from the patient. This is to avoid coercion by the testing center and to support the family members right to decide whether to participate. Blood collection kits along with consent forms are mailed to the necessary family members after the patient provides their names and mailing addresses.

It is optimal to be able to check the family blood specimens for informativeness in the laboratory before collecting blood from the patient. The linkage studies do not work in some families and checking whether they do before drawing blood on the patient prevents the patient from waiting anxiously for results only to hear that no results are available. It also prevents the patient from getting mid way into a costly testing procedure only to find out that they will not receive results.

The total cost to an at-risk individual is about $3000. These costs may increase if a patient is found to need more psychological counseling before testing, or if more than eight family members are needed to provide results in the laboratory, or if the patient must travel a great distance to a testing center.

For the individuals requesting testing, the procedure is time consuming, costly, and emotionally distressing. Most people find this one of the most difficult and important decisions of their lives, underscoring the need for good psychological support and making the counseling sessions an important part of the testing protocol. Most centers employ similar protocols in providing and evaluating this very new type of testing (Huntingtons Disease Society of America 1989).

Ethical Issues Faced When Offering This New Genetic Testing

Several potential ethical issues associated with this type of testing were raised before its inception. However, some unanticipated questions have arisen in practice. In this section, I will discuss some of the ethical questions and conflicts with traditional norms for genetic counseling that have arisen in our experience with presymptomatic testing for Huntington disease.

Beneficence and Nonmaleficence

To provide benefit (beneficence) and minimize harm (nonmaleficence) are foundational goals for health care providers. But questions arise regarding their application in the genetic counseling context.

Should testing be offered to people that tells them about their medical future when there is no known available medical therapy to cure or even slow the progression of the disease? Are we possibly doing more harm than good? Does the potential benefit of knowing one does not have the gene outweigh the potential harm of knowing one does have the gene? Who should decide if such testing should be made available?

We fell back on the foundations of genetic counseling to attempt to answer these questions. We decided the patient is the only one who can truly assess the risks and benefits and that if individuals could utilize this information in their lives, we were obligated to provide it in the best way possible. One of our goals is to provide testing in a manner that ensures informed consent and adequate preparation, while attempting to avoid harm to individuals not psychologically prepared to deal with the results.

Patient Autonomy

Genetic counseling strives to support the patient's self-governance in making health care decisions. However, many individuals say they have experienced a loss of autonomy during the testing and counseling experience. They feel they must convince the testing professionals that they are making a *reasonable* decision *rather* than an informed decision. They sometimes feel the staff is sitting in judgment of their reasons to have the test. Many also fear that to qualify for testing they must have the "right answer" to such questions as, "Have you ever considered suicide?" or "Does your family support you in your decision to have this test?" When a patient or family expresses concerns about the requirements of the testing protocol they are often angry and untrusting. This response interferes with our ability to assess whether they are sufficiently informed and how much support this individual will need if there is an adverse outcome. This raises the question of whether such a testing protocol protects the patient or interferes with their right to have testing?

Our protocol respects the patient's right to make an informed decision by allowing the patient time with appropriate professionals to consider all the implications of their decision. It allows the patient freedom from coercion and supports their right not to have testing after giving them time for consideration. We have found it helpful to discuss our position with the patient during the initial phone contact to hopefully avoid this distressing experience. We also inform the patient that there are no "wrong answers" only answers that can help us provide the best service. If, however, a patient has been diagnosed as having a mental illness or is suicidal, testing will be delayed until psychological staff has determined the individual is not in crisis. An individual in crisis cannot give an informed consent and proceeding with testing under such circumstances may provide the patient with full autonomy but interferes with another primary concern of medicine, that is, first, do no harm.

Confidentiality

Problems of confidentiality abound in presymptomatic testing. If an insurance company is covering the cost of the testing, it is likely to want access to the results. If an employer is supplying the health insurance, it is possible the results will find their way back to the employer. If a family member is contributing a blood sample for testing, they may want to know the results, especially if the results affect their own or another family member's risk. We have encountered challenges from insurance companies and from other family members in our testing experience.

We have chosen to keep patient results in our laboratory only. We will release results, oral and written, to the patient only; if another party (family member, insurance company, private physician, etc.) wishes results they must obtain them from the patient. This places a great burden on the laboratory. The laboratory must develop a system of record keeping separate from the medical center's system and control who has access to these records now and in the future. In the future, with multiple tests available, a different system of record keeping will be required.

Request for Testing from Second Parties

We have received requests for testing from children for at risk parents who do not wish to know their status, from parents of children under 18 years of age, from adoption agencies wanting testing for at risk children for placement purposes, and from physicians wanting testing for individuals who may be showing early symptoms.

We accept only requests for testing from an at-risk individual who is 18 years or older. This position supports the principle of patient autonomy. Autonomy allows an individual control over their decisions about their health care and their future. Conflict does arise when an individual who wants testing needs another family member, who does not want testing, to participate. It is often difficult to identify the patient as genetic diseases usually affect the whole genetic family. We assume the at-risk individual who initiates the testing process is the primary patient.

Less Than Ideal Results

We have had two families whose linkage results were less than ideal. Usually, the linkage results are better than 90% certain. Patients appear to be able to assess these results and utilize them in their lives. In two of our families, the results were 82 and 85% certain. Our dilemma was deciding if these results were informative enough in their predictive value to be useful to the patients. We also wondered how certain they must be for us to say we have an informative family and to report out results.

At this time we have chosen not to set limits on which results we will report out. We have chosen to inform the patient that their results are less than ideal, tell them the percentage of certainty, and allow the patient to decide if the results are useful. The conflict with uncertain results is that we do not want our interpretation of the risk to become the patient's interpretation; however, when the results approach the 50% risk carried by the patient before testing, the test is not very useful.

Family Member Who Refuses to Participate

We have encountered several families where an essential member needed for the linkage study does not want to participate by providing a blood sample. The reasons for this vary. Sometimes one side of the family does not get along with the other side and sometimes a relative feels that no one should have this type of testing. Some patients have requested our assistance in persuading the "uncooperative" individual to participate.

We have placed the burden of discussing reasons for testing on the patient. We supply consent forms and testing information to the patient for distribution to needed family members and remain available to answer questions from anyone in the family. In many cases we do not have direct contact with the patient's family members other than to receive a blood sample and signed consent form in the laboratory.

This position is based on the nondirective objective of genetic counseling. This objective has been questioned in relation to this type of testing. Yarborough et al. published a case study illustrating the conflict between nondirective counseling and the principle of beneficence (Yarborough, Scott, and Dixon 1989). In their case, two family members would not cooperate to help a third member have the test. The third member wished the information for family planning purposes. The authors argue that in some cases it is the counselor's role to do more than provide information and support a patient's decision. The counselor needs to, at times, become directive with a family to fully respect their patient's autonomy.

With our experience, at this time, we do not agree with this position. In some cases this problem can be solved by the counselor offering to call the family member who does not wish to participate and provide accurate information so there is a better understanding of the testing procedure. However, we feel individuals do have the right not to participate in the testing procedure even if their decision interferes with another's ability to have testing. This stance supports everyone's right to make an autonomous decision. Again, this dilemma points out how it is sometimes difficult to know who is the patient.

Prenatal Diagnosis

Whether to offer prenatal diagnosis is a complicated issue. To assure free consent we, along with other centers, have decided not to offer testing to anyone under 18 years of age. However, a woman pregnant with a fetus at risk may wish to have testing to prevent passing the gene on to another generation and subjecting her child to the possibility of inheriting the disease. In some cases women have undergone prenatal testing only to find the fetus has inherited the gene and then decides to continue the pregnancy. This child may then grow up perhaps knowing this information and is not allowed to decide for him/herself whether to be tested. Also, there is the risk that a child known to have the gene may not be treated as "normal."

We offer prenatal diagnosis to women whose pregnancies are at risk. In many families, the availability of this testing allows a couple to have a child knowing that their child will not have to grow up concerned about developing the disease. Some patients have stated that this is one positive use of adverse results obtained on an at risk parent. They feel they are gaining some good from bad much the same way some people feel about donating organs from a deceased loved one. The counseling, however, is in direct conflict with traditional nondirective genetic counseling. We counsel the pregnant woman which prenatal testing is not recommended if she does not intend to terminate a pregnancy involving an affected fetus. Children may be tested later if and when a therapy becomes possible or when they are old enough to make this decision for themselves. We explore with the couple why we do not recommend testing a pregnancy they intend to continue if there is an affected fetus. We are concerned about the burden to the child. Traditional genetic counseling is unconditional, nondirective, and supportive. This counseling is neither unconditional nor nondirective. It is different from the approach used with any other prenatal testing situation and, for me, it makes prenatal counseling for this disease difficult.

Access to Services

Our program is presently one of a few willing to accept patients from all over the United States. Many programs set residency requirements to facilitate appropriate follow-up and will accept only individuals living within close proximity of the center.

We have had difficulty knowing if the families living a great distance from our center have had appropriate follow-up care. The decision not to set requirements for residency was difficult, since we wanted to benefit as many as possible while at the same time avoiding harm to anyone. We decided to offer testing to any individual meeting the requirements of the protocol regardless of where they lived. If a patient comes from a great distance, we ask the patient to contact a local professional able to provide necessary support. If possible, we then work collaboratively with that professional. We feel the principle of justice requires equal access. The most limiting factor for those wanting the test however, is money. For many people, a cost of $3000, and in many cases more, is prohibitive. We therefore do our best to keep costs down and avoid unnecessary visits and tests. Money remains a major issue for us and for most families as it is the foremost factor that limits the allocation of this service. In the absence of a nationalized health care system, finances must be considered in instituting such testing, otherwise the test becomes available only to those who are financially well off.

False Paternity

The possibility of discovering false paternity is a problem with all genetic testing. We have had two families where paternity was a major issue. I will be discussing one of these families in the case study following this section. The ethical conflicts include the patient's right to know if the affected father is indeed the biologic father (meaning if not, the patient is no longer at risk), the mother's privacy right to know that this information will not be divulged, and the father's right to know he is not the biologic father.

Not disclosing the information to anyone. This is one option available, however, it involves an incomplete explanation of test results. For example, if a couple has a child with cystic fibrosis and false paternity is discovered, the "father" may not be a carrier and the couple is not at risk for another affected child. If he separates from his wife and remarries, he may assume he is at risk for a child with cystic fibrosis and choose not to have children with a second wife. If an individual who believes he/she is at risk for Huntington disease has a "father" with Huntington disease, and this man is not the biologic father, the individual is no longer at risk.

This issue is discussed with the patient during the first visit so that if false paternity is a known possibility the patient can inform us and discuss the implications. This was the case with one of our families and preplanning allowed the problem not to become an issue. Also, with prior warning the patient can choose whether or not to know this information should we uncover it during the testing. We also include this information on all of our consent forms so those family members contributing blood samples are aware of this possibility and may choose not to participate. However, since we often do not have contact with other family members, we are unsure if the people giving blood truly understand that this information may be discovered.

Huggins et al. and Morris et al. published articles on the dilemmas and challenges encountered in their experiences with presymptomatic testing for Huntington disease (Huggins et al. 1990; Morris et al. 1989). The issues are similar to those we have encountered in our program. Surely, there are more challenges to come with the arrival of similar testing for numerous other diseases. Our patients and families have taught us much and we are truly grateful to them.

Case Study

This case presented the most difficulty to our testing center. It required an emergency consult from the staff of the University of Minnesota's Center for Biomedical Ethics. It was a disturbing problem because we failed to anticipate it before it occurred.

The wife of a man affected with Huntington disease contacted our center. She stated that her husband had recently been diagnosed with the disease and that her husband's three siblings wished testing. Her husband was eager to help his two brothers and one sister. Both their affected father and unaffected mother were still living and willing to give a blood sample. No other relatives were available. All family members lived out of the state. Testing protocol and cost information were mailed to the individuals requesting testing. We also requested medical records documenting the diagnosis in the affected family members. We waited for them to call and set up appointments.

After a short time, the affected man's sister called and stated that all three of the at-risk family members were interested in pursuing testing and that they wanted to share the costs of the laboratory work. She informed us that money was an issue and that they would be paying for everything out of pocket. We discussed the fact that we would need blood from both of her parents and her affected brother as well as from all those who wanted testing. We also informed her that the testing does not work in all families and that until we tested the blood samples in the lab, we would not know if testing her family worked. We decided to collect blood on all family members and contact her when we knew if results were possible. At that time, travel arrangements and clinic appointments could be made for all who wanted to pursue the testing. She was pleased with these arrangements and supplied us with everyone's addresses. Blood collection kits, testing information, and consent forms were sent to all family members. The laboratory received the blood samples, signed consent forms, and records documenting the diagnosis. Testing took approximately one month. The laboratory then contacted the clinical genetics team asking if there was the possibility of a sample mix up during the blood collection. They stated that their results were unusual and needed review. The family was asked how the blood was collected, telling them that the lab had requested this information. They each had gone to their individual physicians and had their blood drawn and mailed the same day. It appeared there was no chance of a mix up during the blood drawing. The patients were told that we would keep them informed.

Having never come across results like these before, the lab requested that the entire testing group assemble to discuss the possible ways of dealing with the situation. The testing team included a medical geneticist, a genetic counselor, a neurologist, the director of the molecular diagnostics laboratory, the laboratory technologist in charge of Huntington disease testing, the population geneticist who performed the statistical analysis, and a clinical psychologist. This group met with the director and associate director of the biomedical ethics center. False paternity had been confirmed with multiple markers, including other markers than those on chromosome 4 (a VNTR on chromosome 2 and PDP34) in the sister's sample and in the youngest brother of the affected man. The remaining brother was the biological son of the affected father and we could say with greater than 90% certainty that he had not inherited the Huntington disease gene. We discussed the implications and possible consequences of several options. We could (1) tell the family that they were noninformative and results were not possible, (2) tell the family that they were informative and have them travel to our center multiple times to complete the protocol before giving them the results that they did not inherit the gene (do not reveal the false paternity), (3) contact the mother of these individuals and request permission to reveal the false paternity, and (4) have the two people in which false paternity was discovered come for an appointment and discuss the results with them, including the false paternity. We could also ask them what to tell their brother as he needed to complete the protocol. We felt it was necessary for the third brother to complete the protocol in case he demonstrated symptoms on exam. We would then know he had inherited the gene even though the test results showed he most likely had not.

We decided that Option 1 was unacceptable as it would involve lying to the family. Option 2 was also discarded. We felt that this would be deceiving the patient and costly in that unnecessary testing and multiple visits would be involved. Option 3 was a difficult question because by not contacting the mother, she was not given the chance to protect her privacy. However, in the end, we felt that she was not our patient and her right to privacy could not override our patients' rights to make autonomous decisions about wanting the test results. We elected to go with Option 4.

We contacted the sister and told her that the family was informative and set the first appointment. We asked if she and her younger brother were planning to come together for their first visit as they lived in the same small town and in a different state from the rest of the family. She stated that they were planning to come together and that their other brother would be coming later. When they arrived, we reviewed how the test was done and explored their reasons for wanting testing. We reviewed the consent form and discussed the option of not receiving results.

Both were adamant about wanting to continue with the testing stating that they had always wanted to know and now that their brother had been diagnosed they felt they needed this information. The younger brother had recently been married and wanted children if he did not have the gene and the sister wanted to know for the sake of her own two children. We told them the testing had revealed that their affected father was not their biologic father. This would mean that they could not have inherited the gene and therefore could not pass it onto their children. The sister suspected that this was a possibility from family gossip and the younger brother was pleased he would not have children with the disease. They were encouraged to seek professional counseling near their residences in order to help deal with this unexpected information.

The other brother called us later to tell us he had decided not to continue with the testing as he was sure he had the gene. His siblings had called him after they left us and told him their results. He explained that although he desperately wanted to know he did not have the gene for his own children, he feared he would not be so lucky. Again, the testing group contacted the biomedical ethics center for direction. It was decided that we would not be doing any harm and may be benefiting this individual's children if we discussed the results with him over the phone. He was contacted and told that the testing was complicated but revealed that he probably did not inherit the gene. He was given the name of a local geneticist to contact for a genetic counseling appointment. At that appointment he could be educated as to how the test worked and why it was not 100% predictive and what that meant to his family. Results would be discussed over the phone with the geneticist when the patient made the appointment and no written results would be released without a written consent.

Discussion

In our brief experience with presymptomatic testing for Huntington disease, our center has encountered many new ethical dilemmas. Learning how to deal with these issues and, hopefully, predict new ones before they present problems has helped us to refine our procedures so that testing is available to those who want it in a manner that benefits while at the same time prevents harm. In response to the case above, we decided not to take blood from at-risk individuals before visit 3 in our protocol and the lab will not reveal any patient's results until the day before the results visit.

To aid centers in their testing procedures, an ethical issues policy statement has been published by a committee consisting of representatives from the International Huntington Association and the World Federation of Neurology (1990). There are three recommendations in this publication directly applicable to our case: (1) the laboratory should not reveal the test results to the counseling team until very close to the time of the patient's results visit, (2) the test center should not establish direct contact with relatives whose blood is needed for the purpose of testing without the patient's permission, and (3) the possibility of discovering false paternity should not prevent the use of the test.

Although this type of testing is new, it is a preview of the future. With advances in genetic testing, and the information gained through the Human Genome Project, such testing will be available for a multitude of diseases, some of which are very common. The issues will be similar or even more complex. Presymptomatic linkage testing often challenges the foundations of genetic counseling. As discussed previously, genetic counselors are educated to be nondirective and support the patient's values and not allow their own to interfere. This testing has resulted in the need for directive counseling in some cases. Also some conditions have been imposed on the availability of the test and the support the patient will receive. Examples of conditions are: no testing for those under 18 years old and no prenatal testing with the intent to continue a pregnancy when the fetus is found to be affected.

In my experience, I have come to believe that the goals of totally nondirective and totally unconditional counseling are not always possible nor are they always in the best interest of the patient. This testing provides an opportunity to evaluate our goals and values and see where they fit and, in some cases, where they do not work. I feel we are obligated to the public to evaluate this testing and learn as much as possible before it becomes widely available.

One challenge to the genetic counseling profession will be to educate the public about those ethical issues that will affect most people through the development of new genetic testing. Another challenge to the field will be to educate enough genetic counselors to meet the demand for professionals who can facilitate testing for those interested, and who can recognize and deal with ethical problems as they arise.

PART II

---

*Social and Policy Issues in Genetic
Counseling*

Chapter 5

Risk and the Ethics of Genetic Choice

MARC LAPPÉ

Introduction

The essence of genetic counseling is to provide couples with information that allows them to make informed choices about their reproduction. The process of this information giving and subsequent counseling imparts to couples information that ideally enables them to select among diagnostic and reproductive options.

Risk may be of two kinds: *genetic risk,* which is the likelihood of certain genes or chromosomal configurations being transmitted to offspring, and *recurrence risk,* which is the likelihood of the repeat occurrence of a condition in an already born or conceived offspring. Such a condition may have genetic and/or environmental causes. The perception of these risks, singularly or together, and the resultant actions based on these perceptions are subjects requiring careful analysis.

A precise, or more often, approximate risk of an event can usually be calculated based on recurrence estimates, on Bayesian probabilities, and on test outcome. Some of the risks can be intrinsic to the procedure itself (e.g., background risk of miscarriage from "normal conception," chorionic villus sampling, or amniocentesis), while other risks are those generated by the transmission of genetic material and its subsequent interaction with environmental factors during embryogenesis.

Impact of Genetic Counseling

The counseling process impacts on how parents come to view their options and their opportunity for influencing conception or birth. These perceptions often turn on how couples view the risks they are taking for themselves and their future offspring. The subjective element of risk perception governs, in yet little explored ways, a couple's choice to start a pregnancy, elect certain diagnostic tests, and/or abort a fetus. Thus, the "true" likelihood of occurrence of a given outcome (expressed as a probability) may not be as important in certain individual's minds as some other element of that outcome, such as whether or not they can live with a given condition in their newborn child. In this sense, the *perception of* the likelihood of "good" (desired) and "bad" (undesired) outcomes can have as much to do with the impression of a given condition's severity as its likelihood of recurrence.

Risk Perception

People perceive risks based on a complex mixture of subjective and objective beliefs about risk taking generally: the nature of a specific risk, its irreversibility, the likelihood of its occurrence, and the consequences of different outcomes. Other factors, such as ambiguity, control over future events, past experience, and the potentially catastrophic or benign nature of error, are all interwoven into individual risk-taking strategies.

Risk-taking Strategies

Among the biases in risk taking detected by decision-theory researchers are risk aversion, omission bias, and a general bias towards the status quo (Kamm 1986). Risk aversion is the tendency to avoid risk taking, even where it entails accepting a smaller gain than would accrue based on the probability of a desirable outcome if the risk were taken. For instance, people are generally more willing to take a straight cash gift of say $200 than take a 50:50 chance on winning $500.

Omission bias is the tendency to avoid an action rather than committing to one where both actions have the same outcome (e.g., allowing a newborn with anencephaly to die rather than actively killing him). Omission bias is closely related to the tendency to accept the status quo. In the example of the birth of an affected child, omission bias entails passive acceptance of a "fated" future event (i.e., accepting the ongoing consequences of events in progress) rather than taking steps to intervene. Corroboration of this bias can be found in studies of risk-taking strategy: in the absence of definitive information (e.g., about an exact probability that their child is in a group at particular risk of a given adverse event), parents are inclined to withhold action (Ritov and Baron 1990).

The relevance of each of these biases and that they factor into reproductive decision making is self-evident: they predict tendencies toward certain actions when couples face reproductive choices. According to the principle of omission bias, couples will be more likely to hope for the intrauterine death of a congenitally handicapped child than to elect an abortion. Similarly, the existence of risk aversion predicts that couples would refrain from procreation rather than embark on risk-laden pregnancies. And bias toward the status quo predicts that a certain percentage of pregnant women at low or uncertain risk from genetic diseases will accept their fate (i.e., allow the pregnancy to go to term) rather than actively intervene. And, finally, where information is incomplete, couples would be expected not to take any action to change the course of their reproductive decision making.

Decision-making Theory in the Counseling Context

These well-established behavioral norms for human risk taking need to be tested in the often special circumstance of genetic counseling. In counseling, decisions, and perceptions of risk can be skewed by the idiosyncratic and emotionally laden context of reproductive decision making. Decisions about child bearing may differ radically among couples at the same recurrence risk for a disorder depending on their experience (e.g., have they already had a child with a similar disorder), their socioeconomic status; their religious preferences; and the attitude of their doctor toward abortion (Wertz et al. 1991).

Couples at risk for genetic disease may not be risk averse. Nor will they necessarily refrain from reproduction when facing high-risk outcomes, or shy away from risk-laden procedures (e.g., early chorionic villus sampling) if it will give them data on which to act. By definition, few, if any, couples, who seek genetic counseling are biased toward the status quo, since the act of information seeking signals a certain willingness to incorporate new data in their decision making. Most couples would not have elected to seek out genetic advice unless they had some inclination to attempt to understand the consequences of future actions and to alter the course of their reproduction.

Hypothesis Formulation: Characteristics of Genetic Counseling Consumers

The reasons for these trends and attitudes (to be documented below) are sometimes self-evident and at other times obscure. It is my contention that couples who approach genetic counselors of their own volition represent a subsample of the general public in terms of risk taking. They are more inclined toward information seeking or intervention than are others. Couples who have had one affected offspring are more willing to pursue often risky actions to ascertain their genetic status or that of their conceptus, to solicit the aid of others (health professionals, counselors, near relatives, etc.), and to consider abortion (Meryash and Abuelo 1988).

It is also axiomatic that experience, particularly that of having had an affected child, shades choices in the counseling context. Many couples who have still-living children with a given disorder are unwilling to consider selective abortion for a sibling (Markova, Forbes, and Inwood 1979). Thus, the chosen courses of action of genetic counselees will predictably diverge from those of a "typical" cross section of the public.

This is so in part because unexpected and counterintuitive factors can influence decision making in the genetic counseling context that would not necessarily affect more common decisions. For instance, in the mind of the father, the perception of the magnitude of risk from a diagnostic procedure (e.g., chorionic villus sampling) is more associated with maternal occupation and advancing maternal age and education than it is with the actual risk for fetal harm carried by the procedure (Evans et al. 1990). Prenatal choices and risk taking are also heavily influenced by societal forces and expectations. Thus, parents at risk for a subsequent child with a severe mentally handicapping disorder may be more willing to abort a fetus with that disorder than are parents who have a child with a predominantly physical handicap (Beeson and Golbus 1985).

Historical factors may also play a role. For instance, one-third of the Belgian families who believed in the acceptability of terminating a pregnancy where a fetus might be affected with cystic fibrosis had changed their minds between 1984 and 1987 (Evers-Kiebooms, Denayer, and Van den Berghe 1990). The observations suggest that a decision about whether or not to embark on a risk-laden procedure may depend on the perceived impact of choosing or not choosing a particular option, on the stability of a marriage, or on other factors associated only indirectly with genetic risk.

Information Gathering

Couples at risk of transmitting serious disorders tend to be willing to take risks to garner early information about the pregnancy and they tend to elect risk-laden procedures (e.g., chorionic villus sampling) in favor of less risky ones (e.g., amniocentesis) to acquire data about their risk status in time to make a decision to continue or abort the pregnancy. Their willingness to do so is proportional to the risk that the event carries, that is, the higher the risk, the greater the likelihood of allowing early diagnosis (Evers-Kiebooms, Denayer, and Van den Berghe 1990). It is therefore perhaps surprising that in the absence of diagnostic data, couples at risk of having an affected child embark on a pregnancy even where the likelihood estimate of recurrence is high and the disorder quite serious. In one study of 162 couples, 72% of those facing a genetic risk of greater than 15% chose to begin a pregnancy (Frets et al. 1990).

Influence of Experience

It is clear from genetic counseling-generated studies that the perception of risk is also profoundly influenced by past experience. Where couples have previously had a child with a disorder, they are more likely to take steps to avoid a recurrence than when they are naive about such an eventuality (Frets et al. 1990). In the instance of couples at risk for cystic fibrosis, the existence of an already healthy child before the conception of a possible cystic fibrosis-affected sibling tends to discourage reproduction, while more couples are willing to embark on planned pregnancy after having had a first child with cystic fibrosis. This decision is in keeping with the reports in the literature of the negative impact of the severity of disorder on reproductive decisions (Frets et al. 1990).

Beliefs about Severity

The perception of the nature of the recurrence risk that a couple face is also influenced by the impression of what constitutes a "serious disorder." Disorders that are regarded as having a grave prognosis, or where disability is profound are more heavily weighted in decision making than are those that are less serious or potentially treatable.

Other factors that strongly influence reproductive decisions are whether or not other children are living at the time of counseling; the existence of a relative with a similar disorder to the one being anticipated; and, the perception of the likelihood of recurrence.

Risk Taking

Risks are commonly divided by genetic counselors along a gradient of low, moderate, and high risk. By some constructions, these risks correspond approximately to 5%, from 5 to 15% and greater than 15%, respectively. However, families receiving genetic counseling perceive even the choice of language ("low," "high," etc.) and numerical presentation differently. For instance, percentages tend to be perceived as having greater magnitude than do their equivalent proportions (i.e., 10%>1/10) (Kessler and Levine 1987).

Parental age also appears to be a significant variable in risk perception, since being older than 30 (i.e., having fewer pregnancy opportunities) equates with a lowering of the threshold or tolerance for a risk-adverse event. An additional permissive factor in risk taking is nulliparity: couples who did not have children and for whom the occurrence of an adverse pregnancy outcome was interpreted as being 5% or less universally chose to become pregnant (Frets et al. 1990).

This risk factor became even more significant for those couples who already had an affected child. Where genetic diagnosis was available through prenatal testing, half of those couples who had had an affected child opted to refrain from child bearing, while only 14% who were in the identical risk circumstance opted similarly (Frets et al. 1990).

A simplifying form of analysis appears to explain some of this diverse and often inconsistent decision making. According to Lippman-Hand and Fraser (1979), the ultimate choices made by parents are determined by a kind of binary selection between being at risk and not being at risk. In this view, parents anticipate the outcome of events and determine their tolerance to the projected scenario. Hence, the objective probability-based estimate of recurrence times the severity of the disorder becomes subordinated to a simplified analysis in which parents try to live through the prospect of one outcome or the other. Where they find the outcome salubrious and tolerable, they "go with it;" where they cannot live with the outcome (for whatever reason), they try to avoid it entirely (Lippman-Hand and Fraser 1979).

Parents risk-taking behavior is thus a form of loss reduction or minimization, in which the choice of a particular course of action is determined along a bifurcating line between "can we handle this" and "can we afford to avoid this."

Ethical Implications

Because risk is so subjective, several observers have cautioned that counselors may inadvertently (or more rarely, intentionally) skew and influence decision making by the manner in which they present genetic information. For instance, several authors believe that the way in which a problem is presented linguistically or the manner in which it is framed mathematically can have a dramatic impact on decision making. According to one research team, "it is conceivable that counselors might deliberately emphasize one linguistic frame rather than another in order to reinforce or perhaps undermine a decision already made by the counselees." (Kessler and Levine 1987)

The notion that counselors might systematically bias decisions, even as they emphasize their neutral role as information givers, remains an unproven although provocative concept. One reviewer emphasized that "counselors' views may be colored not only by their subjective perceptions of the particular genetic disorder, but also by a tendency to emphasize the social impact of defective children, both as a present burden on health-care resources and as a possible contribution to the future deterioration of society's genetic composition" (Wright 1978).

The willingness or failure to incorporate risk data into a "rational" decision is obviously a value-laden act. Parents are ultimately the persons who must live with their decisions; thereby, the consequences of their actions or inactions regarding recurrence and genetic risks to their offspring. Their children, in turn, carry with them whatever genetically mediated burdens they inherit. Where those burdens are anticipatable it remains a private choice as to whether or not they should be avoided altogether or simply anticipated. Imposing societal views of "acceptable risk" or other constructions of normative behavior is undesirable and unethical relative to the dominant norm in our society of respect for autonomy.

Ethically, decision making is not necessarily less informed or responsible where risks are taken than when those same risks are avoided. However, the proper perception of "risk" will remain a knotty counseling problem unless the counselor understands the context of their clients' risk perception and its social and cultural determinants.

Chapter 6

Discrimination Issues and Genetic Screening

DAN FARBER

Introduction

The New York Times recently reported that a Whittier, California man was denied health insurance because he carried the gene for neurofibromatosis (Blakeslee 1990). As our knowledge of the human genome expands, discrimination of this kind, based on the possession of genetic markers, will become more feasible. Almost inevitably, employers and insurance companies will seek to take advantage of this new knowledge.

The primary purpose of this chapter is to discuss the extent to which these kinds of discrimination are banned by current law. There is no simple legal definition of "discrimination." Instead, the meaning of the term varies depending on which law is under discussion. Thus, rather than a broad conceptual discussion, a careful examination of individual legal rules is required.

The chapter begins with a consideration of the constitutional restrictions on genetic screening. The primary constitutional limitation on discrimination is the Equal Protection Clause. Other constitutional provisions, which are not primarily directed at discrimination, may also be relevant because genetic screening may invade the right to privacy.

The next section turns to statutory limitations on genetic screening. Insurance is primarily regulated by the states and limitations on discrimination are weak. Employment discrimination is subject to federal regulation and some of those statutes may severely limit genetic screening of employees.

Finally, the concluding section of the chapter attempts a somewhat broader perspective. Without attempting a broad philosophical discussion of the ethics of genetic screening, it seeks to identify the primary policies pursued by discrimination law as those bear on genetic screening.

Constitutional Issues

The first question we will address is the constitutionality of genetic screening programs. In considering this issue, a basic limitation on constitutional rules must be kept in mind. In general, these rules apply only to "state action"—that is, actions in which the government itself is in some way implicated. For example, gender discrimination by state government is unconstitutional, whereas gender discrimination by private employers is not. (Of course, there are now statutes that cover most private employers, but the constitutional ban on gender discrimination does not itself apply to them, which is why the statutes were necessary.) In practice, it is often difficult to draw a precise line between purely private actions and those in which the government is implicated. The recent trend of the judicial decisions has been to classify doubtful cases as private, and therefore not covered by the Constitution (Tribe 1988).

The Equal Protection Clause

The Fourteenth Amendment prohibits the states from depriving any individual of "the equal protection of the laws." Despite its brevity, interpretation of this prohibition has sometimes proved both complex and difficult. Plainly, it imposes some requirement of equal treatment. Equally plainly, the law inevitably draws lines and classifies individuals, thereby treating them unequally. Drinking laws distinguish between people on the basis of age, tax laws distinguish on the basis of their sources of income; and family law distinguishes between people on the basis of marital status. The problem, then, is to determine which classifications are permissible, and which violate the constitutional requirement of equality.

The Supreme Court's approach to this problem is to distinguish between arbitrary and justifiable classifications. A classification is justified if it furthers a valid state goal; otherwise, it is arbitrary and discriminatory (Nowak, Rotunda, and Young 1986). But this formulation immediately raises another question: Who is to decide whether a classification furthers a valid state goal—the courts or the legislature?

The answer depends on the type of classification. Some classifications come to court with a presumption of validity; a court will uphold such a classification if it has any conceivable relationship to a permissible legislative goal, leaving it to the legislature to decide the wisdom of the classification. Other classifications are considered presumptively suspect—such as those based on race. With the exception of a small category of affirmative action programs, a racial classification will be upheld only if a court determines that it is necessary to achieve a compelling government interest. Gender classifications belong to an intermediate category, and will be upheld only if they are reasonably related to an important government purpose. This is a stricter standard than most statutes must meet, but looser than the standard for racial classifications (Nowak, Rotunda, and Young 1986).

Where will genetic discrimination fit into this scheme—will it be considered "suspect" like racial or gender discrimination, or will it be allowed so long as it has a rational connection to some conceivable government purpose? In the past, four factors have been important in determining the level of judicial scrutiny: The political powerlessness of the affected group, the prevalence of prejudice or stereotyping, the irrelevance of a characteristic, and the immutability of group membership (Sherry 1984). In general, only the last of these traits applies to genetic discrimination. If a certain gene or set of genes is connected to certain behavioral or biological propensities, the trait is necessarily relevant whenever those propensities are themselves relevant. Thus, genetic traits are not presumptively irrelevant, unlike race or gender. Stereotyping, political powerlessness, and prejudice may sometimes be associated with genetic discrimination, but there is no reason to believe that the carriers of certain genes will be facing any exceptional risk in this regard.

The best indicator of how the courts are likely to rule on the constitutionality of genetic discrimination is the Supreme Court's decision in *City of Cleburne, Texas v. Cleburne Living Center, Inc.* [473 U.S. 432 (1985)]. *Cleburne* involved a local zoning ordinance that required special permission for group homes for the mentally retarded. The Court began with the premise that

> where individuals in the group affected by a law have distinguishing characteristics relevant to interests the State has the authority to implement, the courts have been very reluctant, as they should be in our federal system and with our respect for the separation of powers, to closely scrutinize legislative choices whether, how, and to what extent those interests should be pursued. (473 U.S. at 441–42)

The Court concluded that laws discriminating against the retarded should not be considered constitutionally suspect, and should be upheld whenever they have a rational basis. On examining the facts of the case before it, however, the Court concluded that the ordinance was based on irrational fears rather than on any actual evidence. Hence, it declared the ordinance unconstitutional as applied to the group home in question. If

Cleburne is any indication, genetic discrimination will be allowed so long as it has some reasonable basis and is not demonstrably based on irrational prejudice.

A special problem is presented by genetic traits that are correlated with race or sex. In general, strict judicial scrutiny is triggered only when a classification is either explicitly based on race or sex, or else is intended as a pretext for racial or sex discrimination (Tribe 1988). Hence, the fact that a genetic trait is merely correlated with race or sex will not trigger strict judicial scrutiny, unless the government body was deliberately using the trait as a method of sex or race discrimination. We will see later, however, that a showing of intent is unnecessary under some statutes, although it is required for a constitutional challenge.

Privacy Issues

In our society, privacy has two related but distinct meanings (both of them captured in the phrase, "it's none of your business"). First, privacy relates to certain personal aspects of life that are thought to concern only the individuals involved, rather than the government or other outsiders. Second, privacy is related to the dissemination of information about individuals, which may or may not concern particularly "private" activities.

Fundamental Rights.   The Constitution explicitly marks certain rights as fundamental, such as freedom of speech. Other rights are not given explicit constitutional protection but have been found to be implicit in the Constitution's protection of "liberty" in the Fourteenth Amendment. These rights are often generically described as involving the "right to privacy." Among these rights are those relating to procreation and marriage (Tribe 1988). Genetic screening programs relating to the exercise of these rights would have to pass rigorous judicial review.

In particular, efforts to implement a eugenics program by restricting marriage between carriers of certain traits, or by limiting their right to procreate, would today be considered infringements of fundamental constitutional rights. Such restrictions would be allowed only if a court believed that they were necessary to achieve a compelling government interest. At a minimum, to pass such a test, the trait in question would have to be clearly shown to relate to some disability, and the disability in question would have to be extremely severe. Even then, it is unclear whether such a program would pass constitutional muster. Our experience with compulsory eugenics earlier in this century is a grim reminder of how dangerous such programs can be (Gould 1985). Fortunately, such proposals do not appear to be on the political horizon today.

Testing and the Fourth Amendment. The Fourth Amendment declares that:

> The right of the people to be secure in their persons, houses, papers, and effects, against unreasonable searches and seizures, shall not be violated, and no Warrants shall issue, but upon probable causes, supported by Oath or affirmation, and particularly describing the place to be searched, and the persons or things to be seized.

In construing this provision, the Supreme Court has implied a flexible functional approach that focuses on whether an individual's "reasonable expectation of privacy" has been infringed (LaFave and Israel 1985). In applying this test, the Court has held that there is no reasonable expectation of privacy in a person's facial characteristics or fingerprints, so that it is not a search to observe or record these characteristics. On the other hand, taking a blood sample or using a breathalyzer is a search and therefore subject to the Fourth Amendment (LaFave and Israel 1985). If the Fourth Amendment does apply, a search may or may not be subject to the requirements of probable cause or a search warrant, but the "reasonableness" requirement of the Amendment does apply.

In considering how the Fourth Amendment will apply to genetic screening programs, the best analogy can be found in the Supreme Court's treatment of drug testing. The closest case in point is *National Treasury Employees Union v. Von Raab* [109 S. Ct. 1384 (1989)]. The United States Customs Service requires drug tests, on 5 days notice, for all workers who apply for or who hold jobs that involve drug enforcement, guns, or access to classified material. Positive tests can result in the denial or loss of a customs job, but the test results cannot be turned over to prosecutors without the employee's written consent. In an opinion by Justice Kennedy, the Supreme Court upheld this regulatory program as applied to enforcement personnel.

In a companion case involving railroad workers, *Skinner v. Railway Labor Executives' Association* [109 S. Ct. 1402 (1989)], the Court had concluded that drug testing was a "search" for purposes of the Fourth Amendment, because chemical analysis of urine can reveal a variety of private facts, such as whether a person is epileptic, pregnant, or diabetic. Moreover, the process of collecting urine samples itself implicates privacy interests given our society's attitude toward acts of excretion, while blood testing involves a physical intrusion into the body. Thus, the Fourth Amendment did cover the Customs Service's program.

Justice Kennedy concluded, however, that the warrant and probable cause requirements did not apply to the Customs Service program, so that the only standard was reasonableness. As to individuals involved in enforcement or using firearms, he concluded that the program was clearly reasonable. The government has a compelling interest in ensuring that drug enforcement personnel are physically fit and have unimpeachable judgment and integrity. Moreover, employees who carry guns present a grave risk to the public if they are under the influence of drugs. Their duties involve such serious risks that even a momentary lapse of attention could have disastrous consequences to others. On the other hand, the Court found the evidence insufficient to determine whether the testing requirement for employees handling classified material was reasonable.

Von Raab suggests that the Court will be resistant to compulsory genetic testing. Like urine samples, genetic testing is capable of revealing a variety of private facts about an individual. Genetic testing may involve some physical intrusion such as blood testing, but even if tests are nonintrusive, the disclosure of personal traits is potentially much greater than for conventional blood or urine tests. It seems likely, consequently, that genetic testing will be considered a search for purposes of the Fourth Amendment. If so, it will be subject to a reasonableness requirement. *Von Raab* suggests that the reasonableness standard requires a close fit between the needs of a particular occupation and the trait being tested for. Statistically, drug users probably underperform relative to nonusers (or at least, the Court would probably have accepted the empirical accuracy of this premise). Nevertheless, the Court did not rest on this general statistical observation, but looked for characteristics of various customs jobs that made them peculiarly unsuitable for drug users. The Court focused not only on the relationship between the trait and job performance, but also on the critical public importance of certain aspects of the job. A similar analysis would suggest that genetic testing would be allowed only where a trait is highly relevant to screening individuals who present a serious risk.

A related question concerns the dissemination of genetic information about individuals once that information has been obtained. The Court has been somewhat reluctant to find a constitutional barrier to the dissemination of information, when the collection of the information did not itself invade any expectation of privacy (Tribe 1988). When the Fourth Amendment applies to the collection of the information, however, one element of reasonableness may be the extent to which the information will be kept confidential. Unauthorized public disclosure of personal information might also give cause to tort liability in some states.

Statutory Issues

As we have seen, the Constitution creates some restrictions on genetic screening programs, insofar as those programs are mandated or sponsored by the government. Because of the state action requirement, however, these restrictions do not apply to private employers or insurance companies. Any limitations on private screening programs must be found outside the Constitution, primarily in statutes passed with other forms of discrimination in mind.

Discrimination in Insurance

The insurance industry is almost entirely regulated by state law rather than the federal government. Every state has enacted some form of a model statute governing unfair trade practices, which was drafted by the National Association of Insurance Commissioners. With respect to life insurance, the statute prohibits "unfair discrimination between individuals of the same class and equal expectation of life." As to health insurance, the statute prohibits "unfair discrimination between individuals of the same class and having essentially the same hazard" (Clifford and Luculano 1987). Notice that discrimination is defined here not by reference to broad concepts of fairness, but in terms of actuarial accuracy.

In considering the legality of genetic screening by insurance companies, we may profitably consider the experience with HIV screening. Because HIV testing is plainly related to health risks and life expectancy, the unfair trade statute does not prohibit it as a form of unfair discrimination. In fact, the New York courts have struck down state insurance regulations that prohibited insurers from considering HIV status in writing individual and small group health insurance policies. See *Health Ins. Assoc. of America v. Corcoran* [551 N.Y.S. 2d 614 (A.D. 3d Dept.) aff'd 76 N.Y.2d 995 (1990)]. Essentially, the appellate court held that there was no rational basis for rejecting HIV testing as a sound underwriting practice (Id. at 619). Indeed, one state insurance department now requires insurers to consider applicants' HIV status (Clifford and Luculano 1987).

Some states have enacted special limitations on genetic screening. Massachusetts mandates that insurers provide health insurance coverage for mentally disabled children beyond the age of 19. Other states preclude insurers from denying insurance based on the presence of the sickle cell, Tay–Sachs, and hemoglobin C traits (Schatz 1987).

Under current law, it seems clear that genetic screening is generally permissible, so long as a genetic trait is actually related in a significant way to longevity or health risks. Under those circumstances, to prohibit screening would essentially require that insurance be cross-subsidized at the expense of lower risk consumers. This would present a special problem in the case of individual insurance if the trait in question is usually known to insurance purchasers, since they then have an incentive to buy above-average amounts of insurance. On the other hand, if individual risks can be accurately assessed and discrimination on the basis of those traits is allowed, the risk-spreading function of insurance is gravely undermined (Greeley 1989). At some point, it may become necessary to rethink the role of insurance in a world where detailed genetic information makes risk pooling problematic.

Discrimination In Employment

Unlike insurance, employment discrimination has been predominantly an area of federal law. Since 1964, race and sex discrimination have been governed by the federal civil rights law. Since then, the federal government has also become active in regulating discrimination against the handicapped.

Title VII. Title VII of the 1964 Civil Rights Act deals with employment discrimination on the basis of race or sex. An employer may discriminate in either of two ways. First, the employer may consciously take race or sex into account when making employment decisions. A lawsuit alleging such intentional discrimination is known as a "disparate treatment" case. Second, the employer may use a test or employment standard that does not directly take sex or race into account, but instead has a harsher impact on one sex or race. For instance, a height requirement may be adopted without any thought of discrimination, but it will disqualify more women than men because of the difference in average heights. A lawsuit based on this theory is called a "disparate impact" case. As we saw earlier, the Constitution prohibits disparate treatment by government entities, but not laws that have a disparate impact. Title VII goes farther and prohibits at least some employment practices having a disparate impact (Player 1988).

Since a genetic marker may be much more prevalent in certain racial or ethnic groups, or may be associated with sex, Title VII may be a useful method of challenging some forms of genetic screening. For example, glucose-6-phosphate dehydrogenase is a red blood cell disorder associated with a genetic trait frequently found in African-Americans and people of mediterranean descent (Employment Discrimination 1983:342 n.5). Similarly, the sickle-cell trait almost exclusively affects African-Americans, with an incidence of up to 10%. See *Smith v. Olin Chemical Corp.* [555 F.2d 1283 (5th Cir. 1977)] (rejecting a Title VII claim based on sickle-cell related back disease, where the job involved heavy lifting).

If an employer uses a genetic marker as a ruse for discriminating against a certain group, then the employee has a "disparate treatment" claim. But the employer may be unaware of or indifferent to the sex or ethnic dimension of a trait. In that situation, the employee will have to pursue a "disparate impact" claim.

In *Wards Cove Packing Co., Inc. v. Atonio* [109 S. Ct. 2115 (1989)], the Court made it substantially easier for an employer to defend against such a "disparate impact" suit. Prior to *Wards Cove,* employers had the heavy burden of showing that an employment practice with a disparate impact was required by "business necessity" (Player 1988). *Wards Cove* required only that the employer come forward with some substantial evidence of a business justification, after which the employee then must prove that no business justification exists. Moreover, the practice did not need to be "necessary" for the employer's business; the test was merely whether "a challenged practice serves, in a significant way, the legitimate employment goals of the employer." The employee could win either by proving that there is no legitimate purpose, or that a less discriminatory alternative would serve the employer's interest equally well.

In 1991, Congress amended the Civil Rights Act to overrule *Wards Cove.* Under the amended statute, after the plaintiff shows the existence of a disparate impact, the employer must "demonstrate that the challenged practice is job related for the position in question and consistent with business necessity." As under *Wards Cove,* the plaintiff can also prevail by demonstrating the existence of a less discriminatory alternative. Thus, even if the presence of the marker correlates with race or gender, an employer can lawfully use genetic screening if (a) the genetic marker in fact has a substantial relationship with job performance, (b) no other method of screening would be both effective and less discriminatory.

The Federal Rehabilitation and Americans with Disabilities Acts

The Federal Rehabilitation Act includes two provisions prohibiting employment discrimination against the handicapped. Section 794 prohibits discrimination against qualified handicapped individuals by any federal program or any program receiving federal funds. Section 793 mandates that government contractors take affirmative steps to employ qualified handicapped individuals. These provisions affect approximately 300,000 employees (Employment Discrimination Implications 1983:336). Employees are considered otherwise qualified if they are able to meet all the program's requirements in spite of their handicap; the employer may be required to make reasonable accommodations to make this possible. See *Southeastern Community College v. Davis* [442 U.S. 397, 406, 412–13 (1979)].

In applying these provisions to genetic screening, the crucial question is whether possession of a particular genetic trait qualifies as a handicap. The statute defines a handicapped individual as any person who (i) has a physical or mental impairment which substantially limits one or more of such person's major life activities, (ii) has a record of such an impairment, or (iii) is regarded as having such an impairment. [29 U.S.C. 706(8)(B)(3)]

The critical question facing an individual who has suffered employment discrimination would be whether possession of a genetic marker is an actual or potential "impairment." If the trait has not yet manifested itself, the best argument is that the affected individual is "regarded as" having an impairment by the employer.

The Supreme Court's decision in *School Board of Nassau County v. Arline* [480 U.S. 273 (1986)] supports the argument that individuals who suffer genetic discrimination have a "regarded impairment." Ms. Arline had been hospitalized for tuberculosis in 1957, but the disease was in remission until 1977. After several relapses, she was fired from her job as an elementary school teacher, not because of any physical disability but because of fear of contagion. The Court concluded that fear of contagion, whether or not well founded, was covered by the "regarded impairment" category. The implication seems to be that an individual is regarded as impaired if the employer believes (truly or falsely) that her medical condition presents a risk of inability to meet employment expectations.

Other courts have concluded that individuals with a condition that is not clearly manifested by physical or mental debilitation are covered by the Rehabilitation Act. For example, in *Doe v. Dolton Elementary School* [694 F. Supp. 440 (N.D. Ill. 1988)], the court held that HIV-positive status is an impairment under the Act. On this view, possession of a genetic trait clearly could qualify as a handicap.

The Rehabilitation Act provides substantial protection against genetic discrimination, but its coverage is limited to federally related programs. The recently enacted Americans with Disabilities Act (ADA) expands the employment prohibition to cover private employers [42 U.S.C. 12111(2)]. The new statute defines disability in terms virtually identical to those of the Rehabilitation Act.

The legislative history of the ADA provides strong support for the argument that the statute prohibits genetic discrimination. In discussing the conference committee version of the bill, two members of the House explicitly noted that the ADA protected genetically marked individuals. Representative Owens stated:

These protections of the ADA will also benefit individuals who are identified through genetic tests as being carriers of a disease-associated gene. There is a record of genetic discrimination against such individuals, most recently during Sickle-Cell screening programs in the 1970s. With the advent of new forms of genetic testing, it is even more critical that the protections of the ADA be in place. Under the ADA, such individuals may not be discriminated against simply because they may not be qualified for a job sometime in the future. The determination whether an individual is qualified must take place at the time of the employment decision, and may not be based on speculation regarding the future. Moreover, such individuals may not be discriminated against because they or their children might incur increased health care costs for the employer. [136 Cong. Rec. H; 4614, at 27]

Representative Waxman expressed a similar view [Id. at 35–36].

Proposed regulations have now been issued by the EEOC covering employment discrimination. (Other forms of discrimination are covered by regulations issued by the Justice Department.) The proposed rules define disability broadly and refer to the Rehabilitation Act for guidance. The "substantial limitation" requirement is defined to mean more than the inability to perform a single job. To be substantial, a limitation on employment must include a significant restriction on the ability to perform either a class of jobs or a broad range of jobs in various classes [59 U.S.L.W. 2524 (3/5/91)].

According to the proposed regulations, employers are guilty of discrimination if they (1) disadvantage an individual on the basis of a disability, (2) use discriminatory standards and tests not shown to be job related, or (3) fail to make a reasonable accommodation for an otherwise qualified disabled person. Employers probably will be found to violate the act if they discriminate on the basis of a genetic marker that produces no current interference with job performance, unless the employer can show that there is no practical alternative. If employers must accommodate workers who are currently disabled, they surely should not be allowed to discriminate against a worker based on a mere risk of future disability.

Concluding Thoughts

Genetic discrimination is an emerging problem for both society and the legal system. Undoubtedly, the legal rules covering such discrimination will evolve along with society's attitudes toward the conduct itself. Nevertheless, the legal system already contains the bases for some significant restrictions on genetic discrimination.

As we have seen, the constitutional requirement of equal protection imposes only a mild constraint on genetic discrimination by government agencies. A more serious barrier is probably posed by the Fourth Amendment, which may make it difficult for the government to obtain the genetic information it would need to discriminate. In both the public and private sectors, the most formidable barrier to discrimination may well turn out to be federal legislation protecting the disabled. If possession of a genetic trait is determined to be a disability under those statutes, employers will find it difficult to justify discriminatory treatment. The area in which the legal system currently does the least to restrict discrimination is that of insurance, where any actuarially sound classification is likely to be upheld.

Genetic discrimination raises far-reaching issues of social policy. In general, the legal system has tended to avoid deep philosophical disputes about the nature of equality in favor of a more limited attack on discrimination. Despite their complexity, antidiscrimination laws seem to focus largely on a distinction between prejudice or stereotyping on the one hand, and rational decision making on the other. Thus, the legal system's primary concerns about genetic discrimination are likely to center mostly on questions of rationality, rather than on fundamental theories of egalitarianism.

It will be difficult, then, to challenge genetic discrimination that is based on valid scientific information and sound economic grounds. Nevertheless, even from this relatively narrow perspective, there are two reasons to be concerned about abuse of genetic screening. First, because it is a "hot" new technology, there is some likelihood that genetic screening will become a fad, resulting in overuse. Early studies may contain mistakes or identify traits of limited economic significance, but businesses and government agencies may tend to overestimate the reliability and significance of the scientific results. Second, genetic screening may be linked with existing prejudices about racial groups and gender distinctions. Information that confirms existing stereotypes may be more readily accepted by decision makers, so that implementation of genetic screening may be skewed in a discriminatory fashion. For these reasons, the legal system should at least ensure that whatever genetic screening takes place has a solid basis.

The more fundamental question raised by genetic screening is the extent to which we should define people on the basis of their genotypes rather than their actual behavior or current health. Even in utilitarian terms, it may be rational for individual decision makers to rely on genetic information but irrational for society as a whole. The long-term effect of widespread genetic screening may be to discourage individuals from investing in improving their "human capital." Moreover, even a utilitarian calculation must contend with the fact that we live in a world in which human rationality is far from complete.

Beyond these utilitarian concerns are deeper issues about the meaning of human equality. Our society will be grappling for years with the moral implications of genetic screening. The legal system can make only a modest contribution to the on-going social debate about genetic screening. At least, however, it may be able to prevent some abuses, and to slow the adoption of these techniques to give society more time to respond.

Chapter 7

Role of Public Policy in Genetic Screening and Counseling

PHYLLIS KAHN

The question of how public policy makers should respond to the Human Genome Project is best approached by saying a bit about how politicians respond to important science and technology issues in general (Kahn 1990). As human interactions have increased in complexity and become dependent on more political interaction, science, and technology have become increasingly important to each part of our political system—legislative, executive, and judicial—and at each level of government—federal, state, and local.

"State and local governments employ science and technological knowledge in much the same way as the American populace employs the English language—on a daily basis, unquestioningly and at less than technically attainable standards of performance" (Feller 1980). This statement is also appropriately applied to many elements in both the federal government and the courts.

I am the only elected public official contributing to this volume. This is probably good for the general level of discourse. It should be my role to present a strong defense of our political decision structure. But, although I am a proponent of our system of responsive, representative democracy, I recognize the difficulty in the political consideration of science and technology under such a system.

We are not surprised that the general public feels uncomfortable in areas requiring scientific knowledge, and that politicians reflect this discomfort to an even greater degree. Since their time is often limited and their training is not in these subjects, the pressure of making a wrong decision on some subject they know little about and understand even less appears to be an avoidable risk.

Proponents of special interests take advantage of this discomfort of both the public and the elected politicians. They quickly point out the complexity of the issues and the lack of ability of anyone without years of training in physical, organic, or biomolecular chemistry to comprehend the full ramifications of any such decision. It can be argued that it is better and safer to political bodies to do nothing and to let the experts, that is, the regulatory agencies on one side or the tobacco companies, the chemical companies, or the drug manufacturers, decide.

The scientist, in the public view, takes on conflicting roles. One is that of the neutral technician who merely produces the knowledge and lets others use it. Tom Lehrer (1965) expressed this in one of his songs:

Once the rockets are up
Who cares where they come down?
That's not my department
Says Wernher von Braun.

At the opposite pole are the scientists who think of all knowledge as residing within themselves. The solution then appears to be to find a broker and translator to the public policy makers and in a sense relieve the decision makers of the responsibility of evaluating technical competence. In this simplistic model the best minds are assembled; they ask careful and thoughtful questions, and they reach solid conclusions and resolve the conflicts between any conflicting technical views. The public decision maker then confidently adopts as policy the wisdom so delivered. These are models for the implementation of scientific decisions mainly conceived by scientists and so far unused in the real world as a replacement for the traditional political process. What is actually needed is a level of understanding from both scientists and public officials to effectively intermesh science and technology information and methodology into the traditional political process.

The situation becomes even more complicated for the politician confronted with conflicting scientific advice. Disagreement can occur from basic scientific evidence, from the implications imputed to this evidence, or even from the political orientation of the scientist producing the data. Data can appear to be in conflict just by the means of their presentation; for example, the same number can appear very small when displayed as a percentage of a much larger number or very large when presented as an absolute value. The scale or form of measurement and the intentional use of certain forms of rhetoric can cause confusion. Both the choice of data and the simplifying assumptions used can put a different slant on the final conclusions to be presented. It has been observed (Ozawa and Susskind 1985) that decision makers will give greater weight to scientific advice that supports their personal position and will find reasons to ignore advice that conflicts with their established preference. The existence of conflicting scientific evidence can become the final reason for an official to choose the most politically acceptable conclusion.

We now turn to the public policy aspects of the Human Genome Project. To map and sequence the entire human genome is perhaps the most massive biological project ever proposed by the Federal government. It is expected to cost about $3 billion over the next 15 years with $135 million appropriated in 1991 alone. The funding is divided between the National Institutes of Health (NIH) and the Department of Energy (DOE) and both are required to spend approximately 3% of the appropriation for studies related to the ethical, social, and legal aspects of the project. The involvement of DOE (35% of the budget), an organization comprised mainly of physicists, is a surprise to many biologists, but the connection is in its four national laboratories with the computer power to handle the massive information load of the project (Shoop 1991).

Those who extol the benefits of this project compare it to the Apollo space program (the small step for a man, a giant step for mankind) in its scope and historic significance. They point out the value of improved medical diagnosis, avoidance of birth defects, perhaps even prenatal genetic or medical treatment, the identification of individuals who might be particularly susceptible to specific occupational or environmental disease and more precise forensic practices, already present in the use of DNA fingerprints as court evidence.

Critics of the proposal, however, say that the better comparison might be to the Manhattan Project, and that the ethical, social, and legal controversies could dwarf those that have accompanied the development of nuclear power.

Increased testing and screening for genetic traits have already led to ethical and legal problems. In the 1970s there were some mandatory screening programs for sickle cell trait in black adults and school children that were clearly inappropriately applied. Individuals were turned down for insurance and employment and experienced general stigmatization. Distinction was often not made between the healthy heterozygotes with the trait and those who actually had the disease. At one point the Air Force Academy refused to allow flight training for heterozygotic students (Nelkin and Tancredi 1989).

More recently we have seen a similar issue raised with the question of AIDS testing. The values of confidentiality in the physician–patient relationship, the protection of public health, and the right to privacy may all be in conflict. Decisions now being made in the AIDS arena may be a preview of those to come for human genetics.

The legal and social concerns that might be addressed by political institutions are likely to occur across four areas:

1. medical practice and research
2. employment and the work place
3. the insurance industry; and
4. law enforcement and the courts.

All of these are susceptible to state and federal legislative and executive action. Yet solutions to the problems raised by genetic testing and screening are not necessarily best addressed by law, either legislated or arrived at through judicial interpretation. Often such concerns are handled more effectively by formal or informal standards and private agreements, or professional codes of behavior than by statute or administrative law. With the statement that "We are acting to fill a moral vacuum created by the abdication of the Federal Government" the American College of Obstetricians and Gynecologists and the American Fertility Society have recently established a board to set ethical guidelines for research involving fetal tissue and new reproductive technologies (Hilts 1991).

This action is in response to the truism that any topic concerning sex, even at the level of genes and chromosomes, is automatically controversial, particularly as it might relate to abortion. A news article (Specter 1990) describing the possible cure of a man with Parkinson's disease after a transplant of fetal brain tissue also described the frustration of U.S. scientists who are forbidden by executive order to use fetal material for transplants as long as federal sources of funding support the research. The underlying thought is that somehow the use of fetal tissue will be seen as condoning or even being an incentive to abortion (Tauer 1990). This ban has been continued even though a special panel convened to advise NIH on this issue recommended that federal funds be used for such transplant research (NIH 1988).

This is a particular problem in Minnesota. In recent legislative sessions we have been unable to pass bills updating the state law on organ donation for transplants and research because of the addition of amendments prohibiting the medical use of aborted fetuses (Chandler 1990). A recent positive sign was the nonpassage of any restrictive abortion laws in the past sessions, although all attempts to further liberalize state abortion laws have also failed. A further positive sign on the national level was the passage in Connecticut last year of the first law granting a statutory right to abortion—Connecticut, of all places, the home of the *Griswold v. Connecticut* (1965) decision, where the U.S. Supreme Court was needed to strike down laws restricting dissemination of birth control information and materials.

Expanding on these areas of political interest, first we can examine *medical practice and research:*

When genetic tests become more accurate and available, they will become incorporated into routine medical care. It is also expected that predictive abilities of genetic tests will move much faster than the development of therapeutic or preventive solutions. We will need to answer questions about confidentiality, the status of the doctor–patient relationship, the physicians duty to inform, and the patients access to appropriate counseling.

Some of the particular questions the state must ask in defining its role are as follows:

Will or can a state government protect its citizens from stigmas and labels that may occur as a result of genetic knowledge about individual citizens? Will minority protection laws be needed for them?

What role will or should state government play in protecting individual rights to privacy caused by this new technology? Are these privacy issues the same as other privacy issues, or are there some differences?

What should be the position of the state health and welfare assistance agencies be concerning genetic counseling?

What obligation for health care will/should the state assume once individual new information becomes available about genetic diseases?

Will or should the state take a position regarding the reproduction of persons with known genetic disorders?

Should the state be prepared to pay for the care of these children?

Will the Human Genome Project result in a technology that will permit parents to "order" their baby's physical and mental characteristics, or will/can limits be placed to allow only for the elimination of genes causing diseases or birth defects?

Will less financially advantaged persons be able to participate in the new technology?

Will we end with a "master race" created only by those who are well educated and financially fixed enough to take advantage of a new technology?

In the second area, *Employment and the Workplace,* we have seen genetic and medical screening used to identify workers who may be more susceptible to some substance in the workplace. Will employers be able to exclude such people from certain jobs? A recent Supreme Court decision has just eliminated the practice of excluding women of childbearing age from potentially hazardous workplaces (Petitioners v. Johnson Controls, Inc. 1991).

If genetic testing is used to screen workers at risk for exposure to toxins, radioactive materials, or other biohazards, will employers be required to protect the worker from the risk or face discrimination charges? If genetic screening during the hiring process jeopardizes an applicant's chances because there may be a predisposition for a condition leading to absences, we can pose a two-edged question: First, does state and/or federal law protect such workers from discrimination, and second, are they obligated to inform potential employers of such problems (if they know of them)?

Nelkin and Tancredi (1989) point out that genetic screening is covered by a little known federal regulation (Title XXIX of the Code of Federal Regulators, 1974) stating a requirement for a preassignment physical exam for workers including "a personal history of the employee and family and occupational background, including genetic and environmental factors." The ethical and legal situation is further complicated by the selective distribution of genetic traits and disorders within racial and ethnic groups.

Third, we have the area of *Insurance.* This is one industry that, in its process of risk evaluation is designed to discriminate. Genetic testing results are an obvious tool to establish the risks to the insured parties in a more precise manner. Insurance companies will want to obtain medical data available from genetic screening. They can then use this to set higher rates or deny insurance altogether. If society will not protect individuals from this new menace, Nelkin and Tancredi (1989) warn that "we risk increasing the number of people defined as unemployable, untrainable or uninsurable. We risk creating a biologic underclass."

In the 1991 Minnesota legislative session, a bill (H.F. 2)[2] establishing a limited health care access system was passed. In the section on Health Insurance Reform, Article 7, Section 2, Subd. 2, is a prohibition on health plan companies denying applicants based on "the results of any genetic testing" (JHRSM 1991). Conversation with the sponsor of this part of the bill, Representative Wesley Skoglund, gave further details on this provision. Subdivision 2 is an attempt to eliminate all the unfair reasons for denying insurance coverage, including occupation, age, sex, marital status, race, family medical history, and others. Minnesota is believed to be one of the first states to take this step. The author (Skoglund 1991) reports that the major insurance companies did not object to this provision, possibly because it was a compromise from an original position of *no* ability to refuse. This would have even covered a case where a person suffering a heart attack could stop off at the insurance company for a last minute purchase. It should also be noted that the clause in H.F. 2 does not deny insurance companies the right to reject joiners based on the results of that individual's medical history, including nongenetic tests.

This approach, however, plays down the possible threat to the insurance industry. The availability of information about personal medical risks may allow people to tailor their plan for insurance purchase on their perceived risk. Thus, large insurance policy holders could be only those at greater risk for debilitating and expensive disease.

The wealth of information available from genetic tests may enhance this power to the point that a national government insurance plan or health plan is the only answer.

Finally, the area of *Law Enforcement*.

In the past two years, the DNA fingerprinting technique has been extensively used in hundreds of rape, homicide, and paternity cases. With dramatic claims of its power, the technique was easily accepted in most courts and, with a reputation for infallibility, produced more guilty pleas. It should be noted that the technique is also powerful in establishing innocence, as a false positive match is much less likely than an inconclusive result, should procedural mistakes occur (Fiatal 1990). However, in the pretrial hearings of a case in New York (*People v. Castro*), after objections raised by defense, the evidence was not admitted when the judge ruled that the evidence was not handled properly by the testing laboratory (Neufeld and Colman 1990). Most of the cases where DNA typing was used successfully involved no defense challenge to the evidence.

The Castro case illuminated the difficulties in the technological transfer of a laboratory technique to the more complex street venue of a violent crime. It will most likely result in more rigorous control of standards and both commercial and public laboratories.

The Minnesota DNA Case

Minnesota is a state with legislative and judicial activity in this area. According to the Minnesota Supreme Court's decision in *State v. Schwartz* (1989), DNA evidence is admissible in Minnesota court proceedings if the tests are performed according to appropriate laboratory standards and controls that are sufficient to ensure the reliability of the evidence. However, the court limited the use of DNA evidence in particular cases in two ways: (1) it ruled that the data relied on by the laboratory in performing the test, the test methodology, and the actual test results must be made available to the opposing party before trial for independent review; and (2) it limited the use of "statistical probability evidence" to prove the likelihood of a match between DNA samples, reaffirming a prior decision (State v. Kim 1987). This case involved testimony on blood types where the analyst had concluded that 96.4% of the males in the area (not including the defendant) could be excluded by the test. The court stated that the prejudicial impact of such probability testimony outweighed its probative value, because

> There is a real danger that the jury will use the statistical probability evidence as a measure of the probability of the defendant's guilt or innocence, and that the evidence will thereby undermine the presumption of

innocence, erode the values served by the reasonable doubt standard, and dehumanize our system of justice.

If allowed to stand this is a very antitechnological position, striking at the heart of the usefulness of the high degrees of certainty that may be attained with the proper use of the DNA fingerprinting technique.

In 1989, the legislature enacted language (M.S. 634.26) specifically allowing the admission of statistical population frequency evidence pertaining to genetic markers. This section is designed to overturn the Kim holding, and its outcome awaits a future court case. It is also interesting that the 8th Circuit Federal Court (of which Minnesota is a part) admits such statistical evidence.

Finally, the 1989 legislature directed the State Bureau of Criminal Apprehension to establish and operate a DNA laboratory, requiring the BCA to develop uniform procedures and protocols for the collection of this type of evidence and for the maintenance, preservation, and analysis of the evidence. In 1990 the legislature exempted the establishment of these procedures from the rule-making requirements of the state's Administrative Procedures Act, alleging that the lengthy time required for formal enactment would make it impossible for the BCA to keep up with the rapidly changing scientific developments regarding DNA evidence.

Minnesota's actions are a mini-drama of agency/legislature/court interactions, awaiting a new case for the final or at least the next act. Clearly the court has a go slow attitude concerning this new technology frustrating the agency and the legislature, which are both proponents of its use. Although these events have not had much attention from the general public, there is reason to believe that the public would support liberal use of DNA evidence, in line with other opinions favoring tougher law enforcement. The Minnesota Bureau of Criminal Apprehension (BCA) has just opened the lab and is predicting quicker and more accurate diagnoses than available from the FBI or private labs. In addition they will be keeping a catalog of frozen blood samples from over 1000 Minnesota sex offenders. However, the State Public Defender says that they intend to counter the view that DNA evidence is foolproof and will require money for their own expert witnesses and independent testing (de Fiebre 1991).

For a final summary, in each case we will need to examine current legal policies applicable to genetic testing and screening. We will have to reexamine federal and state statutes, constitutional provisions, case law, and existing professional codes and guidelines. There will be gaps and conflicts in all of these, including public and professional policy. As in any case in which we are dealing with the intersection of science and public and political policy, the solutions are not evident or easy.

The Human Genome Project brings an additional complication with it and that is the ambivalence of the public to abortion. Both the number of abortions performed yearly and the public acceptance of abortions have remained remarkably stable since the mid-1970s with about half the population supporting the current situation (Tauer 1990). Yet the political strength of the antiabortion unit is shown repeatedly in the ban on the use of federal funds for fetal tissue research and the roadblocks put in the way of testing or use of RU-486, the abortifacient developed in France.

Knowledge of the human genome will come with greater ability to detect errors than to correct them. When errors are detected through fetal probes, abortion as the preferred solution becomes much more salient. The problem for ethicists is compounded by the political reality that they may be dealing with an ethic determined by public opinion polling, or even worse, as a reflection of the loudest political vocalizing. The addition of ethicists to the debate through the initial funding stages is positive; but, as one commentator remarked, "The relationship of ethicist to researcher is about the same as that of Army chaplain to general on the eve of an invasion. The ethicist needs to talk to the public, not to the researcher" (Leo 1989). Joseph Fletcher, in his book "The Ethics of Genetic Control," (1988) states:

> We can see that while technology and science solve many human problems they also create new problems in the very process of solving the old ones. To solve these problems we must not and cannot abandon our technology; we have to use more of it. Having bitten into the fruit of the tree of knowledge, we cannot return to Eden. We have reached the end of innocence.

For every academic discipline, human values must be defined in terms of a society whose contours have been shaped by scientific and technological development, a society that we hope has not lost its appreciation of the overriding importance of such human values.

Notes

1. These concepts and related questions are outlined in grant applications submitted to NIH: *State Governments and the Human Genome Project* 1990, submitted by R. Steven Brown, Director of the Center for Environment and Natural Resources of the Council of State Government; and *Ethical and Legal Implications of Genetic Testing* 1989, submitted by Albert H. Teich, Director, Directorate for Science and Policy Programs, American Association for the Advancement of Science.

2. H.F. 2 was vetoed by the governor and did not become law. However, the potential cost of the proposal was at issue; not the prohibition of genetic testing.

Chapter 8

Parables

WALTER E. NANCE

Introduction

The telling of parables has a long history in theology and ethics. Parables illustrate a specific circumstance to which the listener can often relate but may also permit the identification of general principles that can be applied to other situations. So, with apologies to Charles Dickens, I would like to tell you three parables about genetic counseling past, genetic counseling present, and genetic counseling yet to come. The examples I will present are based on my experience with providing genetic counseling for the deaf and for the parents of the deaf.

Genetic Counseling Past

The example of genetic counseling past concerns a couple whom I saw many years ago when I was at the University of Indiana. Their first born child had profound deafness and although there was no family history of deafness or consanguinity, or any unusual features in the child that made us suspect a specific genetic syndrome, we were equally unable to identify any environmental causes such as rubella, prematurity, or exposure to otologic drugs. As is our practice for cases in which we suspect but cannot prove recessive inheritance, we used the empiric risk figure of about 10% as a lower limit and counseled to the couple that their recurrence risk was at least that high, but could be as great as 25%. This couple seemed to be very well adjusted to their son's deafness and were already learning sign language. They very much wanted to have another child but very clearly expressed the view that they did not want to be responsible for bringing

89

another deaf child into the world. I reviewed all the reproductive options that I felt were available then including adoption, artificial insemination, having no more children, or taking a chance but felt by the end of the counseling session that they were really not happy about any of these options. In general, most of the counseling I have given during my career has been at a single session with no systematic attempt to schedule follow-up visits. But in this case, I did happen to see the couple again in a follow-up visit and learned to my amazement and awe that what they finally decided to do was to adopt a deaf child. There is, of course, nothing they could have done that was more in the [self] interest of their own deaf child but they achieved this "selfish" goal without violating their own expressed desire not to bring another deaf child into the world. What has amazed me so much about this case, as I have thought back about it over the years, is how restrictive directive counseling would have been in this situation. This couple found a remarkable solution to their dilemma that was completely outside of my solution set. How wrong it would have been for me by word, deed, or subliminal suggestion to have prevented them from finding their own unique solution.

The other lesson that I have learned from this case is how valuable follow-up contact with families can be, not just for the patients but, in this case, for the counselor as well. Another important dimension of follow-up relates to the transgenerational transmission of genetic counseling. On another occasion at Indiana, I became involved in counseling a large family with X-linked Pelizaeus Merzbacher syndrome, a disease that results in slowly progressive mental and neurologic deterioration. The family had been first diagnosed and studied about 10 years previously and the neurologists who were involved with the family then absolutely could not be faulted in the care with which they counseled the family as to the genetic risk, even to the extent of providing written explanations of the inheritance pattern and risk for relatives. For some reason, this simple information was not transmitted from one generation to the next and when I became involved with the family, another crop of affected males had been born to young women in the family who had not been told that they were at risk. Short of praying for universal health care, which of course would be the answer to many problems in clinical genetics, it is not clear to me that you could design an effective system that would provide the necessary follow-up to prevent tragedies such as this.

Genetic Counseling Present

If follow-up is the parable of genetic counseling past, let me talk now about genetic counseling present. This parable deals with an event that happened during a counseling session several years ago in Richmond. Because of my long-standing interest in hereditary deafness, we frequently see deaf children who are brought by their parents for evaluation. Occasionally we see deaf couples as well who come or are referred to the clinic for genetic counseling. I am ashamed to say that I do not sign and we always employ a professional interpreter rather than a hearing family member for these sessions. One Friday I met with a newlywed deaf couple who were intent on starting a family and had been referred by their physician for counseling. Both the father and the mother were the offspring of deaf parents, and the mother also had a deaf sister. We were able to trace the mother's family history back to individuals who were born before 1900, but were unable to establish any genealogic relationships with the large registry of deafness pedigrees that were collected by E.A. Fay before the turn of the century. Neither parent exhibited any distinctive syndromic features, and it was our impression that both probably had recessive deafness, although it is frequently difficult to be certain even about the mode of inheritance in marriages among the deaf. No other counseling situations are more genetically complex. Because of the high degree of assortative mating that exists among the deaf, pseudodominance can occur and it is not at all implausible that two or more distinct forms of deafness may be segregating within a single sibship. Making use of visual aids and karyotypes, I set about explaining my uncertainty about the alternative modes of inheritance and the impossibility of being certain whether or not they both had the same type of recessive deafness, even if we could be sure their deafness was recessive. I then told them that their risk of having an affected child could be as low as 0 or as high as 100% and that the hearing status of their first child would have an important influence on our assessment of their subsequent risk. I told them that their empiric risk would fall from about 10% to nearly 0% if they continued to have only hearing children and that it would rapidly approach 100% if they only had affected children. I thought I was doing a marvelous job of distilling and interpreting the wisdom I had acquired from 20 years of active interest and research on hereditary deafness. So much so that I scarcely noticed the cloud that had come over the couples faces until the wife plaintively signed through the interpreter "What's wrong with being deaf?"

I suddenly realized how insensitive I had been and how value laden the words I had used were: words like "defect," "abnormality," "affected," "malformation," or "recurrence risk" instead of more neutral terms such as "trait," or "deafness," or "chance" instead of risk. I later realized that this was the first couple I had counseled both of whom were the offspring of deaf parents. Couples of this type seldom seek genetic counseling. The reason for this is that instead of being the ultimate tragedy in their parents lives, the deaf offspring of deaf parents are reared in supportive home environments by parents with whom they could communicate freely from earliest infancy. Is it any wonder that they view their deafness as a defining cultural characteristic rather than a handicap? The couple I was counseling came to the clinic not because of any concern they had about having a deaf child but rather because of their interest in learning about the cause of their own deafness.

After that experience, you may wonder why my colleagues have allowed me to continue counseling at all, much less counseling deaf couples. The truth is, however, that I still do continue to participate in a genetic counseling program for the deaf at Gallaudet University that is directed by a former student of mine, Dr. Kathleen Shaver Arnos. The consulting physicians perform the clinical evaluations and briefly relay their findings through an interpreter to the students who are then scheduled to return for a full counseling session in sign language by Dr. Arnos and her associates. I still slip up occasionally and use the word "risk," but I can always tell when I do it because of the smile that crosses Dr. Arnos' face as she signs the word "chance" instead of "risk."

Genetic Counseling Yet to Come

Now, we come to the parable of genetic counseling yet to come. Human genetics is poised before an era of discovery the likes of which our field has never before witnessed even during the heyday of genetic nosology that occurred in the 1960s and 1970s. It is estimated that the human genome contains somewhere between 50,000 and 100,000 functional genes of which we have some knowledge of perhaps 5,500. This means that by the time the Human Genome Project has been successfully completed at the end of this decade, we will have 10 to 20 times as much clinically relevant genetic information as we do today. At the present time, not a single one of the more than 100 genes that can cause hereditary deafness has been cloned, but a decade from now, they should all have been sequenced. This will pose a difficult dilemma for those of us who are involved in providing genetic counseling for the deaf. It turns out that some deaf couples feel threatened by the prospect of having a hearing child and would actually prefer to have a deaf child. The knowledge that we will soon acquire will, of course, provide us with the technology that could be used to assist such couples in achieving their goals. This, in turn, could lead to the ultimate test of nondirective counseling. Does adherence to the concept of nondirective counseling actually require that we assist such a couple in terminating a pregnancy with a hearing child or is this nonsense? Individuals with whom I have discussed this issue have varied greatly in their responses. Some have drawn an analogy with Catholic physicians who refer patients to other physicians when they require counseling about antenatal, genetic testing. They argued that in the case of a deaf couple, the counseling must be given in the context of, and preferably by, a member of the deaf community. Presumably, such a counselor would share the same values system as the parents and could tolerate autonomy with equanimity. Others with whom I have spoken feel that to assist a deaf couple in having a deaf child would not only be dysgenic but would constitute a perversion of the process of genetic counseling. Still others feel that a consideration of the welfare of the fetus is the key issue and argue that any moral justification that may exist for terminating a pregnancy because of genetic reasons disappears if the fetus is normal.

Just in case you think that this parable of genetic counseling yet to come is overdrawn, I would like to share with you two eloquent editorials that recently appeared in the student newspaper at Gallaudet University that addressed the issue of whether parents should be allowed to use genetic engineering to eliminate deafness in their unborn children. The first student speaking in favor of the proposition wrote:

> I do believe that parents should be allowed to genetically engineer ('gengineer') their offspring in order to remove deafness or other disabilities. Note that I do NOT support the use of gengineering technology to choose gender, race, hair color, or whatever—we speak only of handicaps here.
>
> And deafness IS a handicap, pure and simple, Does anyone really WANT to have to resort to pencil and paper when they try to talk with a non-signing hearing person? To not be able to hear music or announcements made over public-address systems? To be able to use the phone only with people who already have TDDs?
>
> Consider: if the child was to be born blind, or mentally retarded, or crippled, I am certain that all of you would support the use of gengineering to remove the problem. Why should deafness be treated any differently? The negative aspects of deafness are not obvious here, in an environment designed to cater to the deaf, but they ARE real, and when one ventures out into the real world, they make their presence strongly felt.
>
> Those who wish for children to be born deaf to perpetuate the deaf community are selfish. They refuse to consider that the child might want to grow up able to communicate easily with the whole of the country, not just one segment of it. They are so tied to their grandiose vision of deaf heritage that they consider it more important than the rights of the individual. 'I'm sorry, kid, but you HAVE to be deaf. Heritage and all that. I'm sure you understand.'
>
> Using gengineering technology to remove deafness is no more immoral than using a vaccine to cure polio. While we should not feel inferior because of our deafness, neither should we glamorize it to the point where we

consider it an advantage. It is a problem that we can and have overcome, but just because we can live with being deaf doesn't mean that we have the right to force others to be deaf.

The second student was very much opposed to the use of genetic engineering to eliminate deafness and wrote:

> Genetic engineering is mortal man's feeble attempt to play 'God' in order to create a 'perfect child'. Heaven knows how long we've been trying to do this. If it was for the purpose of removing dangerous genetic diseases, mental illnesses, deformity, or the occasional psychopath, I'm all for it. But when it comes to the deafness trait, it stops there. Why would we want to deprive the deaf community from growing? It's illogical and immoral. We're 'asking' for the death of the deaf community, its customs and language.
>
> I'm damn proud of being deaf. Excuse me, I mean Deaf. I come from a very large Deaf family. They've shown me that I can do anything as well as anyone else on this world. They've given me a beautiful language to use, ASL. Have you every watched a young child, perhaps of three to four years of age, using ASL? It's a very thrilling thing to see, something that I never tire of. We have a rich culture, most of it passed down from generation to generation. I don't see anything wrong with being deaf.
>
> Granted, some people will look at us and say, 'You're deaf . . . oh, I'm sorry . . . do you wish you could hear?' Why do those people have to treat us differently? I think the last time I looked in a mirror, I looked just fine. Why do we have to look down on deafness as a curse and disease. Are we any worse off than those who would try to eradicate a whole culture?
>
> I think that being Deaf is a blessing and that's why I vehemently say 'NO!' to the option of removing the deafness gene trait from our DNA. I love being Deaf and I'm damn proud of it!

I think it is clear from these two editorials that educated members of the deaf community are themselves widely divided in their views about the appropriate use of genetic technology. We now know from the varied success of previous genetic screening programs how critically important it is to consider the cultural values of the target population, and it is clear that any program that attempts to provide genetic services for the deaf will have to take these two divergent value systems into account.

PART III

Future Directions and Ethical Challenges in Genetic Counseling

Chapter 9

The Impact of the Human Genome Project for Genetic Counseling Services

HARRY T. ORR

As communicators of information from the medical and scientific communities to individuals at risk for genetic disorders, the role of genetic counselors is directly related to the amount of information available. Thus, programs designed to increase either the pool of information or number of individuals seeking information will expand the role of genetic counselors. The Human Genome Project, or Initiative as it is also designated, is one such program. In fact, the Human Genome Project is very likely the single most influential factor that will affect the demand society as a whole places on genetic counseling services. This increased demand will come from both the medical community and the general population.

The Human Genome Project is concerned with development of technologies for analysis of human DNA. It is also concerned that ethical issues, which arise from an ability to examine the entire human genome at the sequence level, be discussed at all stages of the genome project. Techniques will be developed that may make DNA analysis a routine matter, perhaps capable of being performed in a physician's office. This will likely expand the sites in which genetic counselors will be involved in health care. Hopefully, consideration of the ethical and social issues during the Human Genome Project will help genetic counselors relay the increased breadth of genetic knowledge to individuals and groups so they can deal with the information from a more informed base.

The human genome describes the complete set of genetic information of the human being. The Human Genome Project will progress through three stages, each furthering the precision with which the genome is understood. The goal of the first stage of the genome project is the construction of a genetic map for each chromosome (chromosomes are the chemical packages of genes). Maps of these packages will identify the location of genes within the chromosomes. The genetic maps will be used during the second stage of the project to obtain physical maps of the chromosomes. The final stage involves the cloning of each chromosome. Thus, the last step of the Human Genome Project is the sequencing of some three billion base pairs of DNA, which encompass the entire human genome.

With increasing success, molecular genetic tools have been applied to the localization and identification of genes affected by some inherited disorders. For conditions such as Duchenne muscular dystrophy, cystic fibrosis, neurofibromatosis, fragile X syndrome, and Huntington disease, this technology has increased the precision of information available to individuals from families with these disorders. When the biochemical or physiologic basis of a genetic disorder is unknown, as is presently the case for most human genetic disorders, a sequential, random search of all chromosomes is necessary to locate the affected gene. This search is conducted through linkage analysis. To localize a gene involved in a genetic disorder, normal variations within the human DNA, often called markers, are used. These markers are linked with or located closely to the disease gene on the chromosome. This means that the markers are usually passed on from generation to generation with the disease gene.

By following markers through families, it is possible to identify which individuals have inherited the disease gene. Until recently, the search for disease-linked DNA markers has been random. As discussed previously, the most immediate goal of the Human Genome Project is the construction of a map of the entire genome, which will provide DNA markers evenly spaced along all the chromosomes. This map will be a reference guide onto which a genetic disorder can be placed. Once a gene for a disorder can be located relatively close to DNA markers, carrier testing, prenatal diagnosis, and presymptomatic diagnosis are possible. However, these tests are never 100% certain because linkage analysis follows markers through a family but not directly to the gene.

Although linkage analysis has been helpful for many families, there are limitations. With linkage studies, blood samples are needed from multiple family members, testing is complicated and costly, and a few centers across the country are able to provide the laboratory expertise. This drastically limits access to services for the general population.

The genetic map from the Human Genome Project will provide the basis for the physical mapping and isolating disease genes themselves. Once isolated, a gene can then be characterized to determine the specific mutation(s) that cause the disease. This information makes the direct molecular diagnosis of genetic disease possible. At this point, the results from prenatal, carrier, and presymptomatic tests become absolutely certain.

Direct gene testing will increase availability of genetic testing services. Direct gene analysis requires blood only from the person wishing testing, it is relatively inexpensive, and for many testing procedures it can be adapted to routine laboratory techniques that will increase the number of labs that can provide services.

Once the Human Genome Project enters the third and final stage, the number of disease genes mapped and isolated will surely have increased enormously from the number known today. The third phase will further increase this number as novel genes are identified from analyses of sequence information. More importantly for the discussion here, it is the third and final stage that will likely have the most dramatic effect on the role genetic counselors will have in society.

Through the complete sequence analysis of the human genome novel genes will be discovered, a better understanding of human genetic organization and variation will be obtained, and how a genetic factor impacts human development and behavior will be assessed. Completion of the Human Genome Project could provide information on the role DNA sequences play in the susceptibility to common disorders such as heart disease or hypertension, susceptibility to environmental or workplace toxins, or physical traits such as weight or height. Thus, it is quite likely that many members of society—and not just of families affected with a genetic disorder—will seek genetic information concerning their specific health concerns. Fine (this volume) describes several possible new roles for genetic counselors that may evolve as a result of the information that will become available as the project progresses.

Chapter 10

The Evolution of Nondirectiveness in Genetic Counseling and Implications of the Human Genome Project

BETH A. FINE

To speculate about the future of genetic counseling and its continued adherence to the central tenet of nondirective counseling, a historical perspective of medical genetics and genetic counseling can provide a basis for exploration. In addition, the application of some counseling and ethical theories to the evolving process of genetic counseling must be considered. It has become apparent that the genetic counseling profession has grown concomitantly with the rapid advances in molecular genetics, carrier and prenatal screening techniques, and the increasing understanding of the human genome and its interaction with the environment. New developments in molecular biology and their clinical applications continue to shape the philosophy of genetic counseling and the delivery of genetic services. As the mapping of the human genome progresses, genetic counselors face numerous and complex ethical, social, legal, and educational issues that influence the discipline, the profession, and the daily practice of genetic counseling. An exploration of the impact of the Human Genome Project on genetic counseling as a discipline and a profession, as well as on the values and ethics we embrace, must begin by turning to the past for guidance and insights.

History

Genetic counseling has its roots in the eugenics movement of the early 1900s, which was influenced by the work of Francis Galton. Human genetics, on the other hand, evolved from the concurrent rediscovery of Mendel's laws of inheritance. The discipline of clinical genetics arose from the merging of human genetics and genetic counseling in the medical setting. At the turn of the century, particularly in Europe, many poorly designed studies were utilized to corroborate the notion that social deviants, alcoholics, and the mentally retarded should not reproduce. However, in 1910 the first American "heredity clinic," the Eugenics Record Office, was established by Dr. Charles Davenport in Cold Spring Harbor, New York. This was the first time that scientifically sound genetic research was applied to human genetic diseases to inform individuals and families of genetic risks to themselves or to their offspring. The focus was on the family or individual, not on society at large. At that time, genetic conditions appeared to be rare so that genetics had very low priority in medical school curriculum.

By the 1930s, several factors precipitated the birth of genetic counseling clinics. First, "eugenics" became unpopular as the world witnessed the atrocities in Nazi Germany. Second, as the control of infectious diseases improved, the relative proportion of children with birth defects increased so that medical educators could no longer ignore the discipline of human genetics in their curricula. Third, research geneticists and physicians began to work together; the notion of preventive medicine in relation to genetic disease and birth defects was becoming accepted by the medical community.

Preventive medicine could be considered "eugenic" since the objective is to avoid the birth of babies with birth defects or genetic disease. However, the geneticists in the 1930s and 1940s were proponents of sound scientific research regarding specific diseases. They supported voluntary screening and sterilization. They also believed that, "prospective parents should have access to informed sympathetic counseling when deciding whether or not to have children" (Porter 1977).

Although the term "nondirective" was not yet applied to genetic counseling, the early genetic counselors clearly ascribed to this tenet. In 1947, Dr. Sheldon C. Reed, Director of the Dight Institute for Human Genetics at the University of Minnesota, coined the term "genetic counseling." In his classic book, *Counseling in Medical Genetics*, he defined three requirements for genetic counselors: "some knowledge of human genetics . . . a deep respect for the sensitivities, attitudes and reactions of the client . . . and the desire to teach, and to teach the truth to the full extent that it is known" (Reed 1955). Dr. Reed described his experience with parents of affected children; they never wanted to have a subsequently affected child and often had a strong desire to produce a normal baby. Although he did not use the term "nondirective counseling," the following paragraph indicates that he believed in this value:

they want to know what the chances are of another abnormality. We give them the figure if we have a reliable one; otherwise we tell them that we do not know the value. The parents often ask us directly whether they should have more children. This question is one that we do not answer because we cannot. The counselor has not experienced the emotional impact of their problem, nor is he intimately acquainted with their environment. We try to explain thoroughly what the genetic situation is, but the decision must be a personal one between the husband and wife, and theirs alone. (Reed 1955)

During the 1940s and 1950s, heredity clinics were established at many major university medical centers throughout the United States. In 1948, the American Society of Human Genetics was founded as a scientific and professional organization for clinical geneticists and human geneticists engaged in research. A major goal of the genetic counselors in medical centers was the prevention of birth defects. At that time, the only choice for couples at risk for affected offspring was to reproduce and accept their risk or to refrain from having children. Decisions were called "eugenic" or "dysgenic" based on the chance of perpetuating the condition or gene in the population. The growing experience with the new field of genetic counseling led to an expansion of the scope of the process, as well as the use of multiple disciplines in redefining the practice and the professional training of genetic counselors.

Genetic counseling was originally performed by Ph.D. geneticists engaged in basic science research. Genetic counseling clinics first grew in size and number as a result of the increased clinical applicability of genetic knowledge and as more genetics teams comprised of Ph.D. geneticists and physicians were established (Porter 1977). Eventually, these clinicians could not meet the demands of the clients requesting genetic counseling.

It also became apparent to some clinical geneticists that diagnosis and presentation of genetic risks to individuals, parents, or prospective parents were not sufficient. The psychodynamics surrounding the birth of a child affected with a genetic condition had to be considered by those providing factual information to the parents. Psychiatric research identified the grief reaction after a loss as potentially pathologic, with physiologic and emotional sequelae (Lindemann 1944). In 1961, Solnit and Stark reported that following the birth of a handicapped child, parents experience a mourning process whereby they grieve the loss of the expected healthy child (Solnit and Stark 1961). Despite these and other advances in psychology, the integration of psychology, medicine, and genetics into clinical practice was slow to come, probably due to the absence of multidisciplinary training whereby practitioners could learn to combine these skills and to evaluate the effectiveness of their practices.

A second "explosion" of genetic counseling clinics and an expansion of services occurred in the late 1960s and 1970s, concomitant with the advent of newborn screening for genetic disease, carrier detection, and prenatal diagnosis by amniocentesis. The realization that the population in need of genetic services would grow substantially as more human diseases were found to have a genetic component led to the establishment of the first master's level genetic counseling training program. This innovative program began in 1969 at Sarah Lawrence College in Bronxville, New York, with less than 10 graduates entering the workplace they were destined to create in 1971 (Marks this volume; Rollnick 1984). In that year, the increase in demand for clinical genetic services was reflected in a report from the National Institute of General Medical Sciences. This publication predicted that by 1988, 68% more geneticists would be needed to provide appropriate services (Marks and Richter 1976). Master's level genetic counselors, with their specialized clinical genetic training, were creating their job descriptions and slowly, but surely, filling a necessary niche in the delivery of genetic services.

At the same time that additional graduate programs in genetic counseling were beginning, a shift in emphasis from the prevention of genetic conditions to communication of information to families was taking place among clinical geneticists. Epstein (1975) illustrates this progression in the early 1970s from a genetic counseling goal of the "prevention of genetically determined disorders" to the following definition devised by an American Society of Human Genetics committee in 1974:

> Genetic counseling is a communication process which deals with the human problems associated with the occurrence, or risk of occurrence, of a genetic disorder in a family. This process involves an attempt by one or more appropriately trained persons to help the individual or family (1) comprehend the medical facts, including the diagnosis, the probably course of the disorder, and the available management; (2) appreciate the way heredity contributes to the disorder, and the risk of recurrence in specified relatives; (3) understand the options for dealing with the risk of recurrence; (4) choose the course of action which seems appropriate to them in view of their risk and the family goals and act in accordance with that decision; and (5) make the best possible adjustment to the disorder in an affected family member and/or to the risk of recurrence of that disorder. (Fraser 1974)

Epstein points out that this shift in emphasis resulted, in part, from the fact that the prevention of all genetic disorders is not an attainable goal. Also, it is not appropriate to assume that all at-risk couples feel compelled to prevent a particular disorder. Prenatal diagnosis, for example, is not available for all conditions and is, also, not accessible to all individuals in the population.

Moreover, in a free society, even if preventive measures were possible and available, not all people would voluntarily utilize such services for ethical, moral, religious, or personal reasons. A parent's and society's view of disability and an individual's perception of burden and risk may vary considerably. Therefore, autonomy in reproductive decision making must be preserved in our free society. Questions regarding balancing the ability to treat or manage an affected individual with the options for prevention of the birth of an affected infant have been raised since the concept of prenatal diagnosis arose. These issues have played a role in shifting the goal of genetic counseling toward communication rather than prevention (Epstein 1975).

Additionally, clinical geneticists, trained in the medical model, were beginning to realize that families receiving genetic counseling following the birth of an affected child need more than information regarding recurrence risks and medical definitions. Couples who have terminated a pregnancy after the prenatal diagnosis of a genetic condition need to be prepared psychologically for the sequelae of this difficult decision. The need for a psychosocial component to the "communication process" was becoming apparent to many clinical geneticists. Multidisciplinary training was needed to meet the needs of genetic patients. The "new" master's level genetic counselors found themselves combining genetic knowledge and counseling skills to meet the needs of patients and their families.

Kessler describes a "paradigm shift" in genetic counseling from a eugenics approach to a preventive medicine model and finally to one based in "psychologic medicine" (Kessler 1980). Since the goals of the eugenic or preventive approach could not be achieved, the psychological or communication model became more appropriate. This shift raised important philosophical and practical issues for the providers of genetic services. It became imperative for genetic counselors to receive true multidisciplinary training in the areas of clinical, biochemical, and quantitative genetics, counseling theory and practices, ethics, crisis intervention, statistics, and communication skills. This change, in approach to genetic counseling, led to the need for exploration of issues related to genetic education, decision making, and the genetic counselor's role as supportive counselor and patient advocate while acting as a member of a comprehensive genetic team (Kessler 1980).

As the role of the genetic counselor expanded to meet the growing need for patient care, graduate programs in genetic counseling were being initiated around the United States. In 1974, five programs were in existence. In 1991, approximately 15 programs train nearly 100 students annually. In addition to an increase in the number of training programs, curricula have been revised to incorporate new scientific information and to achieve the specialized multidisciplinary training in psychology, genetics, medicine, ethics, legal and ethnocultural issues, interviewing skills, and public health. An effort to standardize the content of coursework and clinical experience has been made through the National Society of Genetic Counselors (NSGC) and an informal collaboration of program directors. However, the value of diversity in training was recognized as important (Walker et al. 1990).

The NSGC was founded in 1979 with nearly 100 members. This professional organization was established to "further the professional interests of the genetic counselor . . . to promote a network for communication within the profession . . . [and] to deal with issues relevant to human genetics" (Heimler 1980). The NSGC permitted a forum for the exploration of professional issues and an on-going evaluation of the ethics and values inherent in genetic counseling practice. In 1990, a code of ethics was developed for the Society and for its members, with the goal of setting guidelines derived "from principles that would support a value of care and concern" (Benkendorf 1990) (National Center for Human Genome Research 1990). This code of ethics would describe "a set of specific standards of conduct by which [the profession] guides the behavior of its members" (American College of Physicians 1989). This code will facilitate genetic counselors to make professional decisions based on an agreed upon set of minimum standards.

Approximately 1000 genetic counselors in the United States and Canada work in hospitals or university medical centers, while others have expanded their roles into teaching at all levels, counseling in the private sector, laboratory work, clinical research or administration, and into many subspecialties within the field of genetic counseling, such as teratogen counseling or work in a specialty clinic (Baker et al. 1987). As a profession and as individual practitioners, genetic counselors are continuously faced with cases that force us to reevaluate our beliefs and ethical values related to serving our patients.

The Value of Nondirective Counseling

When Sheldon Reed coined the term genetic counseling, the value of nondirectiveness was implicit in his simply stated philosophy. More than 25 years later, the term "nondirective" is absent from the American Society of Human Genetics definition, which is widely accepted by genetic practitioners. The communication/psychological model of genetic counseling asserts that the genetic counselor facilitates an individual or family's decision making by providing unbiased information and assisting them in exploring their own views regarding the available options. For many couples information is desired while prevention by the available means may not be acceptable. One study indicated that patient's reproductive decisions are influenced more by the perceived burden of a condition than by the actual numerical value of the risk (Leonard, Chase, and Childs 1972). Since each individual places his own value on risk and burden, it is generally accepted that genetic counselors should not impose their personal views on patients.

The majority of genetic counselors believe that nondirective counseling is an important goal. While physicians are often in the position to give directive advice, master's level genetic counselors are trained to provide supportive counseling and information that will facilitate autonomous decision making. These counselors might be better equipped to offer nondirective counseling (Powledge 1979). Robert Murray wrote that "the modern definition of genetic counseling clearly states that the counselee will make his/her own decision free of coercion and/or influence of the counselor as is humanly possible" (Murray 1978; Fraser 1979). Epstein (1975) and others have stated that it is not possible for a counselor to be totally nondirective, since nonverbal communication and tone of voice may reveal personal beliefs and attitudes. Patients often ask genetic counselors what they would do if they faced the same situation. The belief in a nondirective ethos leads to a dilemma when this question is posed. This issue has been explored in professional forums at conferences, in the literature, and in graduate program curricula. Most genetic counselors agree that we should not answer this question directly and that we should strive for creating an environment in which the patient feels comfortable making his/her own decision. A survey of medical geneticists in the United States and abroad indicated a consensus that counseling should be nondirective (Wertz and Fletcher 1988a,b; Wertz, Fletcher and Mulvihill 1990). A similar survey of master's level genetic counselors, which has not been done, would most likely reveal similar findings. However, many genetic counselors feel that under specific circumstances, directive counseling may be acceptable and appropriate, when utilized by astute and experienced counselors (Copeland 1989; Godmilow 1990). To understand the basis for the adherence, as well as the deviation from this adherence, to nondirectiveness, an exploration of the philosophical basis for this belief is necessary.

Just as the practice of genetic counseling incorporates skills and knowledge from many disciplines, so have the philosophy and principles evolved in an eclectic way. The commitment to the concept of nondirectiveness is based on the ethical principle of respect for autonomy. Autonomy refers to an individual's right to liberty, to make choices, and to privacy, therefore, the principle of respect for autonomy implies that all people have the capacity to determine their own destiny. The genetic counselor, according to this principle, must treat patients in such a way that facilitates their ability to make choices and take actions based on their personal beliefs and values. Autonomy refers to a person's right to make choices, to privacy, and to freedom (Beauchamp and Childress 1989). The genetic counselor aims to provide comprehensible information in a supportive milieu so that patient autonomy can be preserved as they make reproductive and treatment decisions. Genetic counselors are also guided by the principle of beneficence. Beneficence obligates the counselor to "confer benefits and actively to prevent and remove harms . . . and to balance the possible goods and possible harms of an action" (Beauchamp and Childress 1989). Preventive medicine and public health interventions are examples of societal acts of beneficence. An important goal of genetic counseling is to provide accurate information, presenting the positive and negative aspects of a possible decision, and facilitating autonomous decision making for a patient or family. In practice, individual genetic counselors often focus on acts of beneficence for the patient, family, or, in some cases, the fetus. Conflicts between goals of autonomy and beneficence have and will continue to arise. It is therefore essential to elucidate a framework for ethical analysis for use in individual cases so that practitioners can act in the best interest of patients and their families.

The concept of "nondirective" counseling highlights the value of these ethical principles when counseling patients. In addition to an ethical framework for nondirective counseling, genetic counseling was also deeply influenced by contemporary psychological theory. The "father of Client-Centered Counseling," Carl Rogers, first called his counseling theory "nondirective counseling." Rogers believed that a warm, accepting environment created by the therapist and perceived by the patient as free from pressure or coercion was necessary for successful self-acceptance and self-understanding. In the mid-1940s, Rogers' research in nondirective counseling was driven by the desire to move away from a clinical diagnosis followed by the therapist prescribing a remedy for the problem. In 1951, he changed the name to Client-Centered Therapy to shift the narrower, negative emphasis of "nondirective" to a focus on factors that facilitated client growth (Corsini 1979). Rogers believed that the counselor must communicate empathy, respect, and unconditional positive regard to patients while attempting to "perceive the client himself as he is seen by himself." The counselor should "clarify and objectify the client's feelings" (Rogers 1951). Hence, nondirective counseling does not imply a passive role for the counselor, but one that guides clients in exploration of feelings, issues, and, in some cases, decision making.

The combination of respect for autonomy and the application of Rogers' theory and practice to reproductive decision making forms the basis for the nondirective tenet in genetic counseling. By the time Rogers' theories were adopted, the eugenics focus of genetic counseling was on the wane.

Research has shown that a psychotherapeutic model and a decision making model of genetic counseling consider that the outcome of genetic counseling is not merely the processing of facts. It is generally recognized that facts alone are insufficient for patient coping and decision making (Antley 1979). The psychosocial and ethnocultural context in which information is received and perceived as relevant to a couple or a family is crucial for informed, autonomous decision making. The counselor must present information in a way that is nondirective, yet useful for the patient and family.

In summary, ethical and psychotherapeutic principles as well as a shift from a more eugenic/preventive philosophy to a communication-based model of genetic counseling led to the central tenet of nondirectiveness in genetic counseling. Questions regarding whether or not an individual counselor can be completely nondirective remain unanswered at this time. Some genetic counselors ascribe to the belief that directiveness may be appropriate and beneficial on rare occasions (Godmilow 1990). Despite the inability to resolve these issues in all cases, it is this author's opinion that the value of nondirective counseling is an important one. Genetic counselors must continue to strive for a deeper understanding of their own values and biases in order to preserve nondirectiveness in their practices.

The Future of Nondirectiveness in Genetic Counseling

As the mapping of the human genome progresses, the clinical applications of the new technologies will allow increasing numbers of individuals to face the prospects of genetic testing and counseling. As new genetic information enters mainstream medical practice, provisions must be made for changes in the delivery of genetic services, and potentially, health care in general. This expected increase in clinically useful genetic information will impact on the genetic counseling community and the profession in various ways. The following discussion will explore predictions for the future role of genetic counselors, including professional responsibilities, graduate and continuing education, and mechanisms for dealing with potential clinical, counseling, and ethical dilemmas.

The far-reaching implications of the Human Genome Project stimulate genetic counselors to examine our current priorities and our professional focus. We are challenged to prepare for the future by planning for expected, unexpected, and unprecedented changes in the field of human genetics. Now, more than ever, we must concentrate on our pivotal role obligated to ensure responsible, quality genetics education, counseling and testing with access for all who are interested in these services.

On one level, this is, in effect, a third "explosion" in the demand for genetic services. First, in the late 1960s and 1970s, the advent of prenatal diagnosis for chromosome abnormalities, which was primarily offered to the large group of women of advanced maternal age, led to considerable increases in the number of genetics patients seen as a result of the demand for prenatal testing (Holtzman 1989). Next, in the 1980s, DNA analysis for the diagnosis of disorders such as Duchenne muscular dystrophy and cystic fibrosis, with the possibility of population screening for cystic fibrosis, became available. Genetic counselors were providing services to increasing numbers of individuals who could now benefit from carrier detection and prenatal diagnosis that was not previously available. Genetic counselors faced the challenge of mastery of the intricate principles of recombinant DNA technology in order to accurately and effectively counsel families at risk. These technological advances called for the honing of communication and psychosocial counseling skills as families faced new and difficult dilemmas.

Now, the mapping of the human genome promises an expansion of DNA testing that has significant implications for genetic counseling practice. First, we would expect that virtually all single gene conditions that have serious ramifications for infants and children will be prenatally diagnosable. Hence, the number of patients seeking genetic counseling for prenatal diagnosis of genetic disorders will increase dramatically. These patients will most likely be referred through the "traditional" channels: pediatricians and obstetricians. Well-informed consumers will be referring themselves and making requests based on education through the media. Genetic counselors, however, will be faced with questions regarding the obligation to recontact families seen in the past to advise them of the availability of testing while trying to adequately handle an unwieldy patient load (Andrews 1987). The demand for additional genetic counselors trained at the master's degree level will certainly increase; graduate program directors and the NSGC will need to address this need.

Second, the availability of inexpensive, "routine" DNA testing for disease and disease susceptibility genes for common adult onset diseases such as coronary artery disease, cancer, diabetes, and mental illness will significantly change the role of genetic counselors and the entire genetic services delivery system. For example, if voluntary population screening for disorders such as cancer is offered, health care providers must be prepared to deal with the ramifications of such a program. The reductionist approach of focusing on single genetic results may be in direct conflict with the usual holistic approach of many physicians. Physicians may become confused by the implications of identifying genetic components of certain conditions that were previously thought to be preventable or at least improved by changes in environment or behavior (US Congress OTA 1988). In effect, most members of the population are potential carriers of genes predisposing to a form of cancer or heart disease, for example. Patients must be educated regarding the risks, benefits, and limitations of this type of presymptomatic susceptibility testing. Health care providers will need to help patients decide if they indeed desire the type of information testing can reveal. Informed consent, whether verbal or written, is imperative if beneficence and autonomy are to be preserved. From the legal perspective, case law holds that "competent, adult patients should have the right to decide what is to be done to their bodies" (Andrews 1987). Health care providers will have numerous facts and issues to disclose to patients considering DNA testing. They must also be skilled at psychologically preparing patients for the possibility of positive test results. Health professionals must be knowledgeable about current treatments or behaviors that might ameliorate the outcome. In addition, they must be able to accurately interpret and communicate risk assessment calculations and probabilities to patients. Finally, the health professional must be able to provide emotional support and resource and referral information to patients in need. Most physicians have neither the time nor the training to excel in these and other areas in medical practice. Genetic counselors have the unique multidisciplinary training and experience to assist primary care providers in addressing patient needs.

Most patients who would be offered DNA testing for adult onset disorders would be under the care of internists or family practitioners. These specialists have not traditionally referred to genetic counseling services since little was known or available regarding the genetic component of these disorders. At the current level of staffing, few genetic centers could serve all patients considering this type of testing. A survey conducted in 1985 revealed that respondents anticipated 210 vacancies for genetic counselors and clinical geneticists over the next 5 years (Finley, Finley, and Dyer 1987). I propose that this number will be much higher for the next 5 years considering the expected scientific developments as a result of the Human Genome Project. In addition, a more informed public who are more educated consumers of health care services—as well as a more active mass media—have and will continue to lead to increased genetic referrals.

Manpower issues must be addressed for the long and short term with regard to the provision of genetic services. Genetic counselors are the most appropriate professionals trained to communicate technical and emotion-laden information while facilitating autonomous decision making and adoption of preventive behaviors. Holtzman has written that master's level genetic counselors have the most training in genetics, but that a shortage of these professionals is already apparent (Andrews 1987). The following discussion includes proposals for utilizing genetic counselors to meet the needs of health care providers and patients.

One way to address the shortage of genetic counselors is to expand the opportunity for graduate level training. Recommendations from a meeting of genetic counseling graduate program directors included the establishment of new graduate programs in genetic counseling and to increase the number of students trained annually in existing programs (Walker et al. 1990). Indeed, four new programs have been established in the past 4 years. Some barriers to starting new programs exist with regard to economics in the university settings. Genetic counseling graduate programs are typically small, and do not generate much revenue for the university while faculty, staff, and clinical supervisors must be supported. Nonetheless, new programs will continue to emerge, but the impact on the number of practicing genetic counselors will not be evident for years to come. Most genetic counseling graduate programs are comprised of intensive and extensive clinical experience for trainees. Program directors believe that an increase in the number of students admitted to the programs will compromise the quality of the all important clinical experience due to decreased volume of patients per student (Walker et al. 1990). One option is to have students secure internships at other sites around the country in order to maximize clinical experience.

A second approach to utilizing existing genetic counselors to meet the increasing demand for services is for genetic counselors to assume the role of educator on multiple levels. Public education can be enhanced if genetic counselors work with various forms of media as staff persons or as consultants. Public education by presenting talks to various groups has been an integral part of most genetic counselors' job descriptions (Capra 1989).

Genetic counselors have—and should—continue to contribute to curriculum development and teacher education in elementary and secondary schools, universities, and medical schools (Collins and Schimke 1988; McInerney 1988). Genetic counselors can also educate physicians and other health professionals by participating in and organizing continuing education programs on relevant topics, publishing in professional journals, and consulting with individual practitioners.

Holtzman speculated on the expanded role of the genetic counselor working with physicians who are not geneticists (Holtzman 1989). This could occur on a consulting or on a permanent basis, and might present an alternative to referring all patients in a practice to a genetics center functioning at its capacity. For example, genetic counselors could train physicians and other health professionals to provide pretesting education and basic counseling regarding straightforward or "normal" results. At the same time, these practitioners would be trained to identify those patients who should be referred for genetic counseling. Perhaps an approach to extending the expertise of the genetic counselor is to create a "triage" care setting. This format parallels the delegation of responsibility from clinical geneticists to the "new" genetic counselors in the early years of our profession.

Genetic counselors will also continue to serve as advisors and consultants in university-based and private DNA laboratories. Our expertise in communicating technical information makes us able to serve as the liaison between the laboratory technologists and the health care providers and other genetic counselors.

Genetic counselors must place continuing education as a high priority among professional responsibilities. To that end, genetic counselors must design and conduct research on the effectiveness of genetic counseling and genetics education for patients. We should be developing and evaluating audiovisual materials to increase the number of patients who can be reached with important genetic information. The NSGC must continue to conduct quality educational conferences and publications. We must continue to contribute to a growing body of literature on techniques for handling counseling and ethical dilemmas in clinical practice. The new *Journal of Genetic Counseling*, initiated in 1992, is an excellent forum for such academic and instructional endeavors. Legal, ethical, and policy issues may arise because of the availability of DNA testing resulting from the Human Genome Project. It is possible that mandatory genetic screening for susceptibilities whereby employers and insurers might discriminate to decrease costs to themselves and society will occur, although recent state and federal legislation will preclude potential abuse of these tests. Issues of confidentiality, privacy, and the right to informed consent before testing are but a few areas where a genetic counselor might have impact in responsible utilization of information produced by the Human Genome Project. Genetic counselors might take an active role in the development of public policy by consultation with government officials to ensure the moral and ethical utilization of genetic information with an interest in the individual as well as society at large. These activities in the public arena highlight our role as patient advocates. In short, the genetic counselor has an important role to play in education of the public and professionals at all levels.

The genetic counselor's traditional role as patient–family advocate will continue to be central in clinical practice. Today, we assist families and individuals in comprehending medical and genetic information and in making decisions that are personally appropriate for them. We also assist patients in obtaining services—health care, financial aid, educational programs for handicapped children, respite care—that will benefit their families. I foresee an increase in the scope of this role as advocate as more presymptomatic testing becomes available. Genetic counselors may need to gain knowledge in the areas of estate planning, provisions for living wills, and for skilled care facilities if there is predicted disability, as in the case with Alzheimer's disease diagnosed presymptomatically in a patient's husband or mother. We might be able to advise patients about insurance coverage provisions and employment decisions based on testing for adult onset disease. For example, a patient found to be at increased risk for a certain type of cancer might need support in making a decision regarding leaving a job at which environmental agents increase his chance of morbidity. While we have always facilitated an exploration of options with patients, the scope and number of options will rapidly change considering the results of the Human Genome Project.

In addition to the potential for new, expanded roles for genetic counselors, we must be diligent in promoting and providing appropriate continuing education in new areas. Graduate training in genetic counseling must be continually evaluated and updated to ensure that graduates entering the workforce will be adequately prepared to meet the service demands. The NSGC has and will continue to take an active role in addressing this issue.

The implications of the Human Genome Project for clinical genetics practice extend beyond the practical matters of quality service provision into the area of our philosophy regarding patient care and our professional responsibilities. Can we expect that the availability of new technologies will lead us to challenge our commitment to the value of nondirectiveness in genetic counseling? Are there truly new issues that will arise in our interactions with patients, or will there only be more opportunities for the same types of dilemmas we have always faced? While single correct answers to these and similar questions do not exist, I will describe case scenarios that may challenge an individual genetic counselor's adherence to the principle of nondirectiveness.

Case 1: The Use of Prenatal Diagnosis for Relatively Mild Conditions or Desirable Characteristics

The application of recombinant DNA techniques has made it possible to identify the gene for dyslexia. The researchers who mapped the gene described the benefit of testing for this gene in young children as being the opportunity to identify at-risk youngsters who would benefit from alternative teaching methods. Educational professionals could provide testing and then make recommendations to parents and teachers before the point where the undiagnosed child might face frustration, loss of self-esteem, and ultimately be deprived of an adequate education. However, a patient with several siblings with this learning disability requested genetic counseling to discuss the option of prenatal diagnosis for the dyslexia gene. The patient indicated that she would terminate the pregnancy if the fetus was affected. She stated that she was not willing to see her child struggle in school like her siblings.

Until recently, genetic counselors primarily dealt with the prospect of prenatal diagnosis of life-threatening conditions or seriously disabling conditions. As the ability to test for less serious disorders or even specific characteristics becomes available, many genetic counselors will experience conflicts regarding termination of fetuses with more benign conditions. Genetic counselors must understand their own responses to these situations. Values and perceptions of disorders or "imperfection" change with time, and often reflect societal norms and expectations. Perhaps the definition of "high-burden" and "low-burden" disorders will change with time. For example, several decades ago, individuals with Down syndrome were institutionalized and considered severely handicapped. In more recent years, the benefits of raising a child with Down syndrome at home while enrolling him or her in early intervention infant stimulation programs have become apparent. Semiindependent community-based housing and supervised employment for such individuals have changed society's perceptions of their abilities. Today, many individuals feel they can accept the responsibility of raising a child with Down syndrome, others are certain that they could not. When the burden of the condition is perceived by most individuals, specifically genetic counselors, as relatively low, genetic counselors may feel conflicted about being nondirective. Genetic counselors must be cognizant of societal influences on their own biases and on the beliefs of their patients. The ideal of nondirectiveness should be a goal; conflicts between patient decisions and genetic counselor views should be explored among colleagues when appropriate.

Case 2: Presymptomatic/Susceptibility Testing—a Patient's Choice?

A new test for susceptibility to colon cancer has become clinically available. A couple seeks genetic counselor for prenatal diagnosis because the woman is 38 years of age. The genetic counselor discovers while taking the pedigree that there is a strong family history of colon cancer in the husband's side of the family. The counselor explains the DNA-based test and about the dietary recommendations and regular examinations for early detection. (Data have shown that dietary restrictions and early detection have led to a significant decrease in morbidity and mortality.) The husband refuses to consider testing because he is afraid of finding out he is at increased risk. He is not comfortable with physician visits or testing.

His wife expressed her interest in decreasing his chance of suffering like his relatives. Her husband was firm on refusing testing and preventive measures. Nondirectiveness extends to the need for informed consent to testing as well as for informed refusal. As the Human Genome Project results in technologies that can identify individuals at risk where treatments or preventive measures are available, genetic counselors may face conflicts between respecting autonomy and beneficence. Genetic counselors have counseled patients who choose genetic tests primarily because they are available. The ramifications of not considering the possible outcomes can be devastating for patients. These situations will pose challenges to the genetic counselor who should attempt to present the information in a complete, though unbiased manner. Do we have the obligation to encourage patients to make choices in their best interest? If there is a clear benefit to testing, for example, in order to treat or prevent illness or even death, does nondirectiveness become less important?

Case 3: The Advent of Voluntary Population Screening

Population screening for an α_1-antitrypsin deficiency has become a standard test for all members of the population entering the workforce upon completion of high school or by age 23. Many employers require this test along with preemployment physical examinations. Those patients at increased risk for serious respiratory problems associated with specific exposures in the workplace would be counseled about alternatives to preserve the individual's health and to decrease health care costs to employer. A patient refusing this screening is sent to a genetic counselor.

The genetic counselor must serve as a patient advocate. In accordance with the nondirective tenet, the genetic counselor must consider that nondirectiveness extends to the utilization of informed consent as a vehicle to choose or not choose a test. On a population level, environmentally induced emphysema and cancers can be decreased if preventive measures are taken. All individuals with α_1-antitrypsin deficiency could be identified and directed to safer, lower risk employment environments. Costs, morbidity, and mortality could be substantially reduced. However, the genetic counselor again must respect the choices patients make. She/ he must strive to ensure that the patient is fully and accurately informed, and to exhibit respect for patient's values. Again, the counselor may feel that beneficence may be compromised if a patient chooses to not act in his/her best interest in avoiding illness. In addition, the cost to society versus the individual patient's needs may conflict. Genetic counselors must assess each situation and aim to understand their own views so as to provide effective, unbiased counseling. Sheldon Reed firmly stated that genetic counseling should be conducted considering the best interest of the individual and his whole family, "without direct concern for its effect upon the state" (Reed 1974). Will the availability of population screening for increasing numbers of disease and disease-susceptibility genes force genetic counselors to reconsider this philosophy?

In summary, I submit that the influx of increasing amounts and types of genetic information into mainstream/clinical genetics practice should not alter the genetic counselor's commitment to the principles of nondirectiveness, autonomy, and respect for patients' different values. It is crucial that genetic counselors strive to recognize and accept their own values and ethical beliefs of the profession, while individual genetic counselors work toward understanding their own biases and values in order to provide nonjudgmental, nondirective counseling. Genetic counselors must continue to act as patient advocates and as providers of responsible, quality care. The application of technologies developed as part of the Human Genome Project will drive us to be creative, introspective, and flexible in expanding our roles to meet the genetic and psychosocial needs of our patient populations.

Chapter 11

Objectivity, Value Neutrality, and Nondirectiveness in Genetic Counseling

KAREN GRANDSTRAND GERVAIS

Introduction

Genetic counselors in the United States are almost exclusively guided by the principle of client autonomy in their interactions with counselees (Fletcher and Wertz 1987b). Autonomy requires counselors to remain value-neutral and nondirective in interactions with clients, so that the client's choices are truly expressive of the client's personal values. To maximize client autonomy, the counselor is to provide information, clarify options and their consequences, and assist clients in reaching decisions consistent with their personal values while maintaining a morally neutral posture overall. Thus, the essence of the counselor's role is that of fact provider; the essence of the counselee's role is that of value provider.

This normative model or standard of the ideal counselor–client relation extends a commonly held model of the physician–patient relation into the context of genetic medicine. In this model, decision making is shared and proceeds on the basis of a fact/value division of labor between physician and patient (President's Commission 1983). Applied to genetic counseling, this model permits the genetic counselor to engage in value-based thinking only in a vicarious way, through the values of the client. The counselor is merely an assistant in the process of clarifying and applying the client's antecedently held values to the dilemma genetic information has generated for the client (Caplan, this volume).

That this is the prevailing standard of behavior for genetic counselors is clear in the 1975 statement of the Ad Hoc Committee of Genetic Counseling of the American Society of Human Genetics:

Genetic counseling . . . involves an attempt by one or more appropriately trained persons to help the individual or family to (1) comprehend the medical facts, . . . ; (2) appreciate the way heredity contributes to the disorder, . . . ; (3) understand the alternatives . . . ; (4) choose the course of action which seems to them appropriate in view of their risk, their family goals, and their ethical and religious standards, and to act in accordance with that decision; and (5) to make the best possible adjustment to the disorder in an affected family member and/or to the risk of recurrence of that disorder. (AJHG 1975)

This position is reiterated in the proposed Code of Ethics adopted by the National Society of Genetic Counselors (1991b):

The counselor–client relationship is based on values of care and respect for the client's autonomy, individuality, welfare and freedom. The primary concern of genetic counselors is the interests of their clients. Therefore, genetic counselors strive to:
2. Respect their clients' beliefs, cultural traditions, inclinations, circumstances and feelings.
3. Enable their clients to make informed independent decisions, free of coercion, by providing or illuminating the necessary facts and clarifying the alternatives and anticipated consequences.(National Society of Genetic Counselors)

Dan W. Brock has demonstrated the faulty philosophical bases of any model of shared decision making that presumes a fact/value division of labor between health care provider and patient (Brock 1991). Brock writes:

Although shared decision making is an ultimately sound ideal, a simple physician-patient division of labor between facts and values cannot be plausibly maintained. *One difficulty* is that it appears ultimately still to leave physicians' actions fully under the direction of patients. No more than the consumer sovereignty model does it recognize physicians as independent agents, with moral and professional commitments that can appropriately guide and limit their action in the service of a patient's aims and values. *A second difficulty* is the assumption that, in principle, facts and values can always be distinguished, and in practice can be sufficiently distinguished to permit the physician-patient division of labor.
A third difficulty with the facts/values division of labor is that it assumes that the patient's values or account of the good is correct and so must be accepted and respected by the physician, whatever its content. This is due in part to acceptance of what I have called the extreme subjectivity of values— if a patient's conception of his or her own good cannot be false or mistaken, and cannot be logically incompatible with any facts, then there is no basis for rejecting them as incorrect, false, or unfounded. (Nor is there any basis

for accepting them as correct, true, or well founded, a point commonly overlooked by extreme subjectivists.) (Brock 1991)

The emphasis on shared decision making in the physician-patient relation arose in response to the excesses of medical paternalism and patients' growing sense that treatment decisions reflected values and interests they did not hold. The conviction that treatment decisions should reflect the values and preferences of patients led to the elaboration of a decision-making model that left facts to physicians and values to patients. The beliefs that this division of labor is possible and morally defensible presuppose an untenable view about the differences between facts and values on the one hand (Brock's second difficulty), and untenable ethical assumptions on the other (Brock's first and third difficulties). Brock persuasively diagnoses the root of the error, a mistaken view about the the fact/value distinction itself (which I shall refer to as "the traditional view" throughout this chapter).

This traditional view assumes that our knowledge of facts or objective truths about the world is possible because we are capable of observing nature as it really is: the progress of science, on this view, is progress in perfecting our observational abilities. Values, in contrast, are said to be subjective and dependent on a personal perspective. From this viewpoint there is no way to be certain about values in the way there is to be certain about facts.

If facts and values are as different as the traditional view maintains, then it seems plausible that fact-finding and values-providing are radically different kinds of activities. If they are different kinds of activities, then it may seem warranted, under some circumstances, to assign them to people in different roles. This is the chain of reasoning that connects the traditional view about the fact/value distinction to its associated model of how physicians and patients ought to interact.

All three of the difficulties Brock notes with this medical model apply to genetic counseling. The foundational difficulty with the model is the erroneous assumption that facts and values are logically different kinds of things: facts being the sorts of things associated with objective truth and values with subjective preferences. This view underwrites a particular normative model or standard for the activity of genetic counseling. This normative model, in turn, informs a particular conception of how medical professionals ought to participate in decision making with patients, and how genetic counselors ought to engage themselves in clients' decision-making process.

Epistemology, a view about what constitutes knowledge, underwrites ethics: A fact/value division of labor between a health care provider and a patient–client presupposes a distinction between facts and values; a fact/value distinction presupposes a particular view of objectivity. But, this conception of objectivity has been criticized and rejected by contemporary philosophers. If any of these challenges to the fact/value distinction are compelling, value neutrality in genetic counseling must be rejected. Rejecting the features of the traditional view entails rejecting the understandings of autonomy, value neutrality, and nondirectiveness that presuppose a fact/value distinction.

After summarizing the revisions urged on us by contemporary philosophers concerning the nature of objectivity, facts, and the fact/value distinction, I shall comment on the impacts of these revisions on the ethical duties of the genetic counselor. These revisions require corresponding revisions in the traditional understanding of the genetic counselor's duties to clients—not so much in what those duties are, but in what constitutes their performance.

"Facts" and "Values"

John Stuart Mill distinguished facts and values, science and art, in this way:

> Science is a collection of truths; art a body of rules, or directions for conduct. The language of science is, This is, This is not; This does, or does not, happen. The language of art is, Do this; Avoid that. Science takes cognizance of a phenomenon, and endeavors to discover its law; art proposes to itself an end, and looks for means to effect it. (Mill 1874)

Mill implicitly characterizes science as the paradigmatic value neutral activity, and articulates the fact/value distinction. The assumption that a fact/value division of labor between counselor and counselee is possible presumes that facts and values are distinct in principle and distinguishable in practice. Three formulations of the opposing view that facts and values are distinct in principle *but not distinguishable in practice* have appeared in recent philosophical work. For the sake of convenience and clear reference, I shall refer to these three attacks on the traditional view as the science argument, the ethics argument, and the language argument.

The science argument stresses the practical interdependency of facts and theories. The ethics argument sees all human activity (including science) as determined by the interests and values of those wielding social and political power. Each of these arguments attacks the traditional view's conception of scientific objectivity and provides a distinct set of grounds for viewing pure science (e.g., the mapping of the human genome) and any derivative activities (e.g., genetic medicine and genetic counseling) as theory dependent and value laden. Their common claim against the conception of facts as free-standing, observer-independent entities is that facts are contingent, observer-dependent entities.

The science argument locates the contingency of facts in their theory dependency; the ethics argument locates their contingency in the value dependency of theories. In addition, the ethics argument includes an ethical/political analysis of the origin of the traditional view's theory of science and objectivity itself. The science and ethics arguments maintain that theories and concepts (the science argument) and values (the ethics argument) are the necessary prerequisites for the human activity of determining facts. Thus, while facts are distinct in principle from their underlying theories and values, they always come "attached" to both theories and values.

Recent arguments in philosophy of language focusing on the nature of language and communication also undermine the traditional view. Since genetic counseling is essentially a communication activity, the language argument that a fact/value distinction cannot reliably be observed in the practice of communicating suggests that the duties of communicating in value neutral and nondirective ways require substantial explication.

While these three arguments are very different in character, they are similar in outcome. Each in its own way undermines the claim that the counseling relationship can be established on the basis of a fact/value distinction, and thus forces a redesign of the model of shared decision making and a redefinition of its duties. The science argument demonstrates this model's reliance on a naive view of facts, theories, and the nature of science. The ethics argument accuses it of failing to note the respects in which the distribution of power in and among cultures determines what is valuable, what theories are pursued, how knowledge is sought, and, ultimately, what counts as knowledge and objective truth. The language argument points to the practical impossibility of purging evaluation from the activity of communication itself.

The Traditional View and the Science Argument

Archimedes, that he might displace the whole earth, required only that there might be some one point, fixed and immovable, to serve in leverage; so likewise I shall be entitled to entertain high hopes if I am fortunate enough to find some one thing that is certain and indubitable.

René Descartes

On principle it is quite wrong to try founding a theory on observable magnitudes alone. In reality, the very opposite happens. It is the theory which decides what we can observe.

Albert Einstein

The traditional view considers science the domain of objective truth because scientific judgments are verified by observation. It presumes that there is a privileged perspective from which scientific claims are "properly" to be tested and verified, that the scientist can adopt this proper perspective, and that this perspective is in fact the one adopted by the scientist in distinction from other commentators on reality. Thus, it affirms that the Archimedian point Descartes yearned for exists, that knowledge is possible, and objective truth is attainable.

Recent work in epistemology, philosophy of science, and philosophy of the social sciences has called this understanding of objectivity into question, in effect saying that the Archimedian point is where for prevailing cultural reasons it has been put. Going back to Archimedes and his desire to move the earth, this position would advise him that there is not just a single special point at which to put his lever, but a number of possible points. While he might not have been able to move the earth equally or to the same new location from all of these points, he would have been able to move it at least somewhat and in some "direction" using any of them as his point of leverage.

The key criticism of the traditional view centers on the claim that observation, and thus the identification of facts (i.e., scientific truths) is theory dependent. Our descriptions of reality are constructed from within a theoretical framework of concepts and laws: the framework is the condition that leads us to see what we see and to describe its relationships to the other things we see as we do. While the traditional view claims that observation is the foundation of scientific theory, Einstein claims that theory provides the context for observation and the reporting of facts. Hence, theory precedes and founds observation.

Contrary to the traditional view, then, the science argument has an alternative philosophical perspective on the connection between observation and theory construction in science. The traditional view assumes that there is an observational stance that discloses nature to us as it is. Thus, the growth of science is made possible, indeed is entirely dependent on, enhancing human powers of observation to render the previously unobservable observable.

By contrast, the science argument holds that observation occurs in a context: the theory we embrace sets the terms of observation. Our theory is often transparent to our view because it plays a role in the identification of facts analogous to the role played by corrective lenses of eyeglasses in vision: theory is the perspective we have inherited for viewing nature accurately, and, thus, is the condition of vision that does not itself fall within our visual fields. Unless we consciously attend to it, it is for all practical purposes invisible to us. The understanding of the notion of objectivity or objective truth that follows from this view of the theory dependency of observation is that truth is context dependent. It requires the careful naming of the place where one stands, the correction values of the lenses one is wearing, to fully describe nature on this view.

Some see the above dispute as the death knell of any workable concept of objectivity. They conclude that the theory dependent character of observation renders all observations relative. They deny that there is any security in the tentative Archimedian points Einstein implicitly identified as the birthplaces of all scientific strivings.

Others come to more hopeful conclusions, believing that the notion of objectivity can and must be analyzed to reflect the theory-dependency of observation. The point of scientific striving is to be clear about one's stance, to have a pragmatic justification for it, and then to engage in meticulous observation and inference from within that perspective (Brown 1987). Such an approach admits that objectivity is not to be equated or identified with certainty. It emphasizes a more modest view of knowledge. It emphasizes the character of scientific observation as a continuous interaction with the natural world, an interaction the character of which permits the scientist to work alternatively with the assumptions of the authoritativeness and the tentativeness of well-tested theories.

The Traditional View and the Ethics Argument

> The search has been for an approach to the real on which to base arguments and conclusions that will make one's point of view unquestionable and unanswerable, immortal and definitive and the last word, regardless of time, place, or person . . . Its history is the history of an attempt to exert such power over reality as comes from methodological hegemony over the means of knowing, validating only those ways of proceeding that advance the project of producing what it regards as requisite certainty. Objectivity has been its answer, its standard, its holy grail. When it speaks and there is silence, it imagines it has found it.
>
> Catherine MacKinnon

The ethics argument goes beyond the science argument in two ways. In agreement with the science argument on the theory dependency of observation, it points to the value basis of all the theory choices that are made. Then, as a specific application of this more general insight, it locates the emergence of the traditional view (and its attendant concept of objectivity) in the value perspective constituted by the experience of the powerful—in Catherine MacKinnon's case, men.

The ethics argument identifies objectivity as a value-driven presumption, reflective of the interests of the powerful in maintaining their position of social and political power. However, this view sees the search for the Archimedean point as a search that would be undertaken only by those holding a particular value perspective on nature. It identifies the notion of objectivity itself as a conceptual construction that could have been invented only by those consistently holding the dominant position in the social order. On this view, theories and concepts reflect the political/moral structure of human society. A particular conception of knowledge and truth originated out of a moral and political situation of inequality. The resulting ideology has become a central, pervasive tool for maintaining the unequal distribution of political power by disguising evaluations as facts.

This attack on the notion of scientific objectivity goes beyond the science argument in locating the emergence of the concept of objectivity in a particular value perspective. It points to the value dependency of all of the theoretical choices we make. The ethics argument examines the processes of theory choice and concept formation themselves. In agreement with the view that observation is theory dependent, it takes the further step of arguing that these activities are a function of the prevailing values of those in power in a particular society.

The primary contemporary source of this critique of the concept of objectivity appears in feminist philosophy; some feminist thinkers locate the view of nature implied by this notion of objectivity in male political power. Objectivity itself is declared to be a male norm, formulated from the standpoint of a faulty moral and political experience that has yielded a jaded value stance toward nature. If this attack on the notion of objectivity is correct, it suggests that scientific activity, insofar as it instrumentalizes nature and other humans, represents a normative choice that must be continuously evaluated for its moral and social–political impacts. It suggests that there is no such thing as the value-neutral "doing" of science (Harding 1986; Warren 1987).

The Traditional View and the Language Argument

The traditional view embodies a claim about language. It holds that facts and values are distinguishable in practice to such an extent that a value-neutral science is possible. The corollaries of this view of science are that value-free language and value-free communication are possible. A duty to be value neutral in one's communication with another assumes that there is a way to use language that is value neutral.

This view of language has been called into question on two grounds that are especially relevant to a consideration of the duties of the genetic counselor to be value neutral and nondirective. The first is that the meaning of language is inextricably tied to collateral information, information that contributes evaluative content to it. The second is that speech acts between persons may acquire evaluative content through their performance by particular persons, and/or their occurrence in particular contexts (Root forthcoming).[1] Neither of these arguments demonstrates that it is in principle impossible to excise evaluation from the language passing between persons, only that there is never any guarantee that this has been achieved in practice.

The philosopher W.V. Quine has argued that there are no clear lines along which to distinguish the meaning of language from the beliefs members of a given community hold about it (Quine 1960). Words cannot *predictably* play a simply descriptive function because of the collateral information associated with them in the minds of both speaker and hearer. To the extent that collateral information is evaluative, the use of language is evaluative. Since the meaning of language is inextricably linked to the beliefs of language users, actual communication between persons relies on a sharing or identification of surrounding beliefs, some of which are inevitably evaluative in character.

Another argument states that communication between persons easily roams from description to prescription due to the context of the communication, the roles of the communicators, and the interpretive frame the hearer imposes on the "facts" presented. G.P. Grice and J.L. Austin have attended to the "pragmatic facts about the use of an expression in a language" (Root 1992). They maintain that particular utterances by particular persons in special contexts are unavoidably evaluative. The question this analysis raises for constructing a normative model for genetic counseling is whether, and if so how, the context of genetic medicine, the counselor–counselee relation, and the sorts of utterances made in the counseling process unavoidably carry this evaluative weight. The traditional view assumes that with the appropriate sorts of effort language can be kept in a pristine value-neutral state, thus permitting purely descriptive communication between persons. On the view of communication just described, this view is not compelling (Grice 1975; Austin 1975).

Conclusion

I have developed three lines of philosophical argument that question the concept of objectivity and the fact/value distinction associated with the traditional view. The prevailing normative model in genetic counseling recommends a fact/value division of labor between counselor and counselee that presupposes the traditional views of the fact/value distinction and its underlying concept of objectivity. The counselor provides the factual basis for the client's decision, while the client provides and applies values to those facts to reach a decision.

Three philosophical objections to the fact/value distinction undermine any model that recommends a division of labor along fact/value lines. How do they require us to rethink the genetic counselor's duties to promote autonomy and to interact in a value-neutral and nondirective manner with clients?

First, the assumption that the counselor can engage in value-neutral communication must be replaced by the assumption that some evaluation necessarily attends this specialized communication with another. Specifically, the interaction between counselor and counselee occurs within a layered context of human activity that includes science, genetic science, medicine, and genetic medicine. Each of these carries with it particular theoretical and value commitments, all of which culminate in a particular concept of genetic health and disease. This concept dictates which options are labeled and presented to counselees as "medical" options. The science and ethics arguments indicate that a number of theory choices have been made at each level of the layered context within which genetic counseling occurs, each theory choice derived from prevailing values, each of which has brought us to our present cultural/historical juncture. At this juncture, genetic counseling is increasingly conceived as a standard medical role.

A skeptic might argue that genetic counseling is a political rather than a medical pursuit, and thus that genetic counseling is being falsely sheltered under the umbrella of medicine. This skeptic might call our attention to the findings of some who have surveyed the habits of genetic counselors both nationally and worldwide and have found that counselors overwhelmingly favor a highly individualistic conception of client autonomy, even failing in some instances to impose a concept of health and disease on client choices based on genetic information (Fletcher and Wertz 1987b). Thus, the skeptic might say, "Better to regard genetic counseling as a family-design or social engineering pursuit. Putting it under the medical rubric legitimates the analysis of the human being it allows, and enables decision making that is not even arguably about disease."

Although one need not subscribe to this extreme position, one cannot avoid noting that since the human body and its characteristics are the subject of analysis, the assumptions that we must be "doing science," and "doing medicine" in all activities derived from that science, is a view that reflects a particular theory of what medicine is, possibly an outmoded theory in the era of genetic medicine. It is clear that a series of theoretical and value choices has generated the practice of genetic medicine, and exerts evaluative impacts on the genetic counselor's determination and presentation of facts and options.

Since one is not engaged in a value-neutral activity, due to the layers of evaluation and choice that have given rise to it, the pertinent issue for the genetic counselor becomes the extent to which central theoretical and value commitments are shared by the counselor and counselee. The realization that the fact/value distinction is a myth requires the counselor to make reasonably certain that the counselee grasps and accepts the central values governing their encounter.

Second, a particular (medical) concept of genetic health/disease determines the genetic counselor's selection and presentation of facts. The genetic counseling literature has demonstrated that counselors and clients may differ in this concept (Sellars). Thus, special attention to producing clarity in the counselor's and the client's concept of genetic/ health and disease is essential, since it influences the counselor's determination of the facts that constitute relevant information for the client's decision. The counselor is not achieving an appropriate measure of value neutrality in the presentation of facts if that presentation is not based on an awareness of the client's concept of health and disease. But insofar as genetic medicine enables clients to consider positive eugenic goals (e.g., increasing height, intelligence) and not simply negative ones, negotiation (over and above clarification) of the operative notion of health/disease may be necessary between counselor and client.

Third, the possibilities created by genetic medicine undermine the acceptability of a blanket principle of patient autonomy, most commonly grounded in the claim that since the patient must live with the outcome, the patient's values ought to ground the decision. It is often the case in genetic decisions that the client is not the only one who must live with the outcomes of the decision. The pursuit of genetic medicine thus requires a rethinking of the meaning of the principle of autonomy.

The appropriate conception of autonomy may require that a client's decision be made in light of a full appreciation of all the ramifications of choice, including the outcomes it will have for others and the values those others would be likely to place on those outcomes (Yarborough et al. 1989). Since genetic decisions may be morally far reaching in ways that standard medical decisions are not, one of the implications of exploding the fact/value distinction is that the sorts of decisions made possible in genetic medicine require that the concept of autonomy be dislodged from its individualistic moorings and be given a more communitarian spin. The resulting revision in the conception of autonomy will be that autonomy is enlarged by knowing what one is doing, not by doing what one wants. Such a revision in the meaning of autonomy will require the counselor to direct the client through a much more intensive values-based scrutiny of the available options, playing an active role in expanding the client's awareness of the evaluative issues posed.

While a thorough-going values scrutiny is a directive activity, it is not value-directive in the sense that the traditional norms of genetic counseling sought to eliminate. Instead, it directs the client to contemplate the full extent of the value dilemma. If autonomous choice on the part of clients requires the counselor to play a far more values-conscious role, the education of genetic counselors must include the careful nurturing of normative reasoning skills. Rather than making a mockery of the notion of nondirective interaction with clients, these skills will enhance the counselor's capacity to convey options and the values they promote, more firmly setting the stage for clients' critical assessment of their situation, their values, and their consequences.

Such nondirective interactions require special skills on the part of the counselor, skills at discerning all the relevant arguments and assisting the client in exploring their value dimensions and their logic without directing clients to a specific decision. These are preeminently philosophical skills. The training of the genetic counselor should involve in depth training in ethical analysis and critical thinking. If it is unreasonable to add this additional element to the education of genetic counselors, it may well be essential to bring someone into the counseling interaction who does have these skills in values elucidation and argumentation.

The three philosophical challenges to the fact/value distinction cut deeply against the grain of the prevailing model that has informed the genetic counseling role. The untenability of this distinction, and thus the untenability of dividing labor along its lines, forces us to rethink our understandings of the central duties of the genetic counselor.

If the ethics argument is right, there is no such thing as value neutrality. If the science argument is right, all the activities that have led to the development of the genetic counseling role presuppose theory choices that are based in values. These theoretical and value beliefs cannot be purged from our communication with each other, but they can be identified, brought to conscious awareness, and subjected to moral reflection. Thus, the counselor's duty is to promote as much clarity as possible about the values that condition the presentation of facts and options, and the values that are at stake in the client's choice. To assist the client in a full awareness of these factors is to enhance rather than to narrow autonomy.

Note

1. Professor Root's manuscript was particularly helpful to me in developing this brief characterization of the language argument for the purposes of this chapter.

Chapter 12

Ethical Obligations of Genetic Counselors

LEROY WALTERS

This chapter is divided into four parts. First, I will present three ethical principles that are widely regarded as important within the field of biomedical ethics. Second, I will indicate how one of these three principles is generally accepted as the predominant principle in the traditional ethic of genetic counselors. In the third part of the chapter, I will explore how an ethic that gives primacy to respect for autonomy is already being challenged by some hard cases for genetic counselors. The fourth and most speculative part imagines how future technological or social developments could raise additional challenges to the predominant view.

Three Ethical Principles

In the work of two national commissions and a widely used textbook on biomedical ethics, three ethical principles have been identified as quite important: beneficence, justice, and respect for autonomy (National Commission 1978; President's Commission 1983b; Beauchamp and Childress 1989). The first of these principles, beneficence, is also called well-being or welfare in the broad sense. The principle of beneficence focuses our attention on the benefits and harms of an action or policy. In other words, this principle asks us to look at the consequences, outcomes, effects, or utility of what we do. (Some commentators, including Beauchamp and Childress, have distinguished a principle of nonmaleficence, or not harming, from the principle of beneficence (Beauchamp and Childress 1989). In this analysis, I will include the notion of not causing harm within the broad concept of beneficence.)

The principle of justice also has multiple names. Some commentators prefer to use the terms equity or fairness. This principle looks first and foremost at how the benefits and harms covered by the principle of beneficence are distributed. There is a formal principle of justice that almost everyone can subscribe to—namely, that every person (or living being) should receive his or her (or its) due. However, various theories of justice disagree vigorously on just how we should determine what is due to every person or living being (Beauchamp and Childress 1989). It should also be noted that some philosophers apply their theories of justice not only to the distribution of harms and benefits, but also to the liberty rights that are often derived from the third principle, respect for autonomy (Rawls 1973).

Respect for autonomy also goes by other names. It is often simply called liberty or respect for persons. Some philosophers would limit the coverage of this principle to persons, a subset of human beings who possess a minimum level of intellectual capability (Engelhardt 1986). Others argue that at least higher nonhuman vertebrates are capable of a certain type of autonomy that ought to be respected. The principle of respect for autonomy is frequently made more specific through the assertion that the persons or other beings who deserve our respect have certain liberty rights.

My personal view is that the three principles of beneficence, justice, and respect for autonomy are helpful in analyzing ethical decisions or the policies adopted by professional groups or public policy makers. The three principles do not, in my view, exhaust the categories that can be applied to decision making or policy making. However, the principles can serve as a kind of checklist, or points to consider, in ethical analysis. If we take the three principles into account, we are probably less likely to make a serious moral mistake than if we omit one of the principles or, more radically, ignore the principles altogether.

Some philosophers have argued that in cases of conflict among the three principles, one of the three should always take precedence over the other two, or even that there is an order of priority among the three principles. Thus, some utilitarians argue that the net benefit of an action or policy should be our primary concern. In contrast, most egalitarians would argue that maximizing net benefit is less important than equalizing welfare—insofar as possible. Libertarians and other proponents of individual liberty assert that achieving net benefit or producing equality of welfare is less important than respecting the free choices of persons. My own view, in consonance with that of Beauchamp and Childress, is that it is impossible to discover or justify priority making among the three principles that is relevant to all situations (Beauchamp and Childress 1989). In other words, our judgment is always required, and any one of the three principles may take precedence in a particular case or with a specific policy.

The Traditional Ethic of Genetic Counselors

In this part of the chapter, I will not attempt to break new ground or to make controversial claims. Rather, I will simply report on what seems to be generally accepted about the predominant ethos among genetic counselors. In its influential 1983 report on genetic screening and counseling, the President's Commission on Bioethics noted the high priority that postwar genetic counseling has placed on respect for the autonomy of clients (President's Commission 1983a). This approach was based in part on a rejection of the coercive eugenic policies that had been employed in the United States and Nazi Germany earlier in the twentieth century (Reilly 1991; Proctor 1988). It was also indebted to Carl Rogers' notion of client-centered therapy (Rogers 1951; Reed 1974; Fine, this volume).

Dorothy Wertz and John Fletcher have recently documented the extent to which the principle of autonomy takes precedence over other ethical principles among one group of genetic counselors, medical geneticists. In their responses to 14 clinical cases, medical geneticists from 18 countries cited the principle of autonomy as their first or second reason for their answers 59% of the time. The consideration cited next most often, the principle of nonmaleficence ("not harming"), was cited only 20% of the time. The principle of beneficence ran a distant third at 11%, while the principle of justice was appealed to in only 5% of the responses (Wertz and Fletcher 1989).

There are two primary implications of the principle of respect for autonomy in the genetic counseling relationship. The first is that genetic counselors are generally committed to respecting their clients' freedom to make their own decisions. The second is that genetic counselors have a strong commitment to protecting the privacy of their clients and the confidentiality of information about the lifestyles or genetic conditions of those clients.

Current Challenges to the Primacy of Respect for Autonomy

In an effort to determine under what circumstances the principle of respect for autonomy might be called into question in current practice, I have chosen the following strategy. Wertz and Fletcher conducted a 19 country survey of 682 medical geneticists between June 1985 and February 1987 (Wertz and Fletcher 1989). One of the researchers' findings was that 3 of the 14 clinical cases included in their questionnaire had proven to be the most difficult to resolve, both for medical geneticists in other countries and for those in the United States. These cases, in decreasing order of difficulty, concerned (1) prenatal diagnosis for sex selection, (2) the confidentiality of information about a Huntington's disease patient, and (3) the disclosure of false paternity (Wertz and Fletcher 1989). I hypothesized that these cases might have been ethically difficult precisely because they presented challenges to the dominant ethic of respect for client autonomy. Thus, I needed to look both at the respondents' answers to the questions and at the reasons they gave for their answers.

Case 1

The case about prenatal diagnosis for sex selection, question 12 on the survey instrument, was framed by Wertz and Fletcher (1989) as follows:

12. A couple request prenatal diagnosis for purposes of selecting the sex of the child. They already have four girls and are desperate for a boy. They say that if the fetus is a girl, they will abort it and will keep trying until they conceive a boy. They also tell you that if you refuse to do prenatal diagnosis for sex selection, they will abort the fetus rather than risk having another girl. The clinic for which you work has no regulations prohibiting use of prenatal diagnosis for sex selection. What would you do?
    1. grant their request for prenatal diagnosis
    2. refuse their request for prenatal diagnosis
    3. try to dissuade them from having prenatal diagnosis, and if they still insist on having it, refuse their request
    4. refer them to another medical geneticist or genetics unit offering the service
    WHY did you select this course of action?

The responses to this question by 295 U.S. medical geneticists (74% with M.D. degrees, 22% with Ph.D. degrees, and 4% with other advanced degrees) follow (n=292; there were 3 nonrespondents):

	Value	Frequency	Valid (%)
Perform diagnosis	1	94	32.2
Refuse to perform	2	54	18.5
Dissuade, then refuse	3	56	19.2
Refer	4	83	28.4
Dissuade, perform	5	5	1.7

The principal reasons for their answers given by U.S. medical geneticists, in descending order of frequency, were the following (for principal reasons given by more than 5% of the 275 respondents who provided one or more reasons):

	Frequency	Valid (%)
I do not approve	70	25.5
Right to decide—parents	44	16.0
Use resources wisely	37	13.5
Prevent harm—child	27	9.8
Don't abort normal fetus	26	9.5

The responses to the same question by 387 non-U.S. medical geneticists were as follows:

	Value	Frequency	Valid (%)
Perform diagnosis	1	66	7.0
Refuse to perform	2	105	27.1
Dissuade, then refuse	3	186	48.1
Refer	4	29	7.5
Dissuade, perform	5	1	0.3

The first reasons given for their answers by 5% or more of the non-U.S. geneticists were the following, in descending order of frequency (331 provided first reasons):

	Frequency	Valid (%)
I do not approve	75	22.7
Don't abort normal fetus	66	19.9
Use resources wisely	59	17.8
Prevent harm—child	26	7.9
Right to decide—parents	18	5.4

These results indicate that 32% of the U.S. medical geneticists surveyed would perform prenatal diagnosis for reasons of sex selection; an additional 28% of geneticists would refer the couple to another provider that offers the service. In contrast, only 17% of non-U.S. geneticists would perform prenatal diagnosis for this indication, and only 8% would refer. Only two other countries had as high a percentage of medical geneticists who would perform prenatal diagnosis for sex selection as the U.S. did— Hungary (60%; $n=15$) and India (37%; $n=27$) (Wertz and Fletcher 1989).

The principal reasons given by respondents reflect appeals to diverse ethical principles. The concern to respect the autonomy of the prospective parents, who were viewed as the principal clients, loomed much larger among U.S. geneticists than among their counterparts abroad. The prevention of harm to the potential child is a reason derived from the principle of beneficence (or nonmaleficence), and the admonition to use resources wisely seems to be based on the principle of justice. Two other reasons are not easily related to the trilogy of ethical principles. The simple statement of nonapproval seems like a straightforward conscientious refusal to be an accomplice in an act that is judged to be morally wrong; another way to interpret the nonapproval reason is as an implicit request that clients also respect the autonomy of health professionals. The reason "don't abort normal fetus" is open to a variety of interpretations. It could be an appeal to the proper role of a geneticist—treating or preventing disease—or an implicit protest against unfair discrimination on the basis of gender.

Case 2

The case concerning the confidentiality of information about a Huntington's disease patient, case 2 in the survey instrument of Wertz and Fletcher (1989), was formulated as follows:

2. A client recently diagnosed as having Huntington disease (HD) refuses to permit disclosure of the diagnosis and relevant genetic information to siblings who may be at risk for Huntington disease. In your professional capacity as a medical geneticist, what would you do?
   1. respect the client's desire for confidentiality
   2. provide the information to siblings, whether or not they ask for it, only after all reasonable efforts to persuade the client to consent to voluntary disclosure have failed
   3. provide the information to siblings only if they ask for it, and after all reasonable efforts to persuade the client to consent to voluntary disclosure have failed
   4. provide the information to siblings, taking care to ensure that only information directly relevant to the relatives' risks is provided, regardless of client's desire

5. provide the information to the client's referring physician, and let that physician decide about disclosure

WHY did you select this course of action?

The responses to this case given by 295 U.S. geneticists were the following (*n*=289):

	Value	Frequency	Valid (%)
Respect confidentiality	1	114	39.4
Tell relatives	2	24	8.3
Tell sibs only if they ask	3	82	28.4
Tell sibs relevant information	4	45	15.6
Refer info to patient's doctor	5	24	8.3

When they were asked why they had responded as they had, U.S. geneticists gave the following as their principal reasons (*n*=274):

	Frequency	Valid (%)
Right to know—relatives	71	25.9
Right to privacy—patient	71	25.9
Duty to warn third party	37	13.5
Doctor–patient relationship	31	11.3

The responses to the same question given by 387 non-U.S. geneticists were as follows (*n*=383):

	Value	Frequency	Valid (%)
Respect confidentiality	1	104	27.2
Tell relatives	2	37	9.7
Tell sibs only if they ask	3	146	38.1
Tell sibs relevant information	4	55	14.4
Refer info to patient's doctor	5	41	10.7

The first reasons given for their answers by non-U.S. geneticists were the following (*n*=332):

	Frequency	Valid (%)
Right to know—relatives	115	34.6
Right to privacy—patient	63	19.0
Duty to warn third party	40	12.0
Doctor–patient relationship	26	7.8

These results indicate that 39% of U.S. medical geneticists would preserve patient confidentiality in this case, whereas only 27% of non-U.S. geneticists would. Conversely, 62% of non-U.S. geneticists would disclose information about a Huntington's disease patient's diagnosis to the patient's relatives, while only 52% of U.S. geneticists would. The major difference among those willing to disclose was the relatively larger proportion of non-U.S. geneticists willing to respond to a request for information by the patient's relatives (38% vs. 28%).

A close examination of the principal reasons given for these answers indicates that the right to privacy was assigned higher priority by U.S. than by non-U.S. geneticists. This autonomy-based right was cited by 26% of U.S. geneticists but by only 19% of geneticists from other countries. The principle of beneficence (or nonmaleficence) probably underlies appeals to the relatives' right to know and the physician's duty to warn third parties. By a margin of 47% to 39%, non-U.S. geneticists were more likely to make these appeals than were their U.S. counterparts.

Case 3

The third difficult case for medical geneticists involved an incidental finding of false paternity. Wertz and Fletcher presented this case as follows (Case 5):

5. You are evaluating a child with an autosomal recessive disorder for which carrier testing is possible and accurate. In the process of testing relatives for genetic counseling, you discover that the mother and half the siblings are carriers, whereas the father is not. The husband believes that he is the child's biological father.

Would you
1. tell the couple what the laboratory tests reveal about the child's parentage
2. tell the couple that they are both genetically responsible
3. tell the couple that the origin of the child's disorder is not genetic

4. tell the couple that you have not been able to discover which of them is genetically responsible
5. tell the couple the facts about the child's parentage, and try to get the name of the child's biological father so he can be told that he is a carrier
6. tell the mother alone, without her husband being present

WHY did you select this course of action?

Among U.S. medical geneticists, the responses to this case were as follows (*n*=288):

	Value	Frequency	Valid (%)
Don't mention results	0	1	0.3
Tell couple all	1	12	4.2
Say both genetically responsible	2	19	6.6
Say don't know which responsible	4	3	1.0
Tell all, find biological father	5	4	1.4
Tell mother alone	6	241	83.7
Give risk of 25%	7	1	0.3
Say new mutation is cause	8	7	2.4

When asked why they had responded as they had, U.S. geneticists cited the following reasons as their principal considerations (*n*=273):

	Frequency	Valid (%)
Preserve family unit	103	37.7
Right to decide—patients	45	16.5
Honesty, tell truth	15	5.5
No need to know	14	5.1

When asked about this incidental finding of false paternity, non-U.S. geneticists provided the following answers (*n*=383):

	Value	Frequency	Valid (%)
Don't mention results	0	2	0.5
Tell couple all	1	12	3.1
Say both genetically responsible	2	44	11.5
Say disorder not genetic	3	4	1.0
Say don't know which responsible	4	12	3.1
Tell all, find biological father	5	0	0.0
Tell mother alone	6	304	79.4
Give risk of 25%	7	1	0.3
Say new mutation is cause	8	4	1.0

The first reasons given for their choices by non-U.S. geneticists were the following (*n*=332):

	Frequency	Valid (%)
Preserve family unit	132	39.8
Right to decide—patients	45	13.6
Right to privacy—patient	36	10.8

In their responses to the false paternity case, an overwhelming majority of both U.S. and non-U.S. geneticists (84% and 79%, respectively) opted to tell the mother alone about the incidental finding, in her husband's absence. The next-most-frequently chosen response, in the U.S. and abroad (7% and 12%, respectively), was to tell the husband and wife that they were both genetically responsible—an assertion that was contrary to the facts as reported in the case at hand.

The first reason cited by a plurality of both U.S. and non-U.S. geneticists for their answers was a consequential reason—the desire to preserve the family unit. This reason was cited by 38% of U.S. geneticists and 40% of geneticists from other nations. Note that this reason could have been used to support virtually any of the responses except the two "tell all" options. The appeal to this reason could envision one or more possible harms—the breakup of the marriage, the rejection of the child by the husband, or physical injury that might be inflicted by an angry husband on either his wife or the child or both. The outcome orientation of this reason clearly identifies it as beneficence (or nonmaleficence) based.

Slightly less important, both in the United States and abroad, were reasons that seem to be based on the principle of autonomy. The reason "right to decide—patients" seems to imply that the mother should have the discretion to decide how much to disclose to her husband. Similarly, the "right to privacy" seems to refer to the woman's interest in keeping information about the child's true paternity from her husband. These reasons were cited as the most important reasons by 24% of non-U.S. geneticists and 21% of U.S. geneticists (if one includes the 4.8% of U.S. geneticists who appealed to the right to privacy). Respondents gave much less emphasis to another possible application of the autonomy principle: only 6 of 605 respondents in the United States and abroad asserted that the spouse had a right to know in this case.

From the analysis of these hard cases based on the current practice of genetic counseling I draw two conclusions. First, what makes these cases difficult is in fact the conflict of the principle of respect for autonomy with other principles, as well as the problems that occur if traditional autonomy-based rules are rigidly followed in certain circumstances. At the level of the principles, we have seen that respect for autonomy is relevant not only to the client but also to the counselor. We have also noted that a couple is not a single person and that respecting the autonomy of each member of a couple may involve the counselor in difficult moral quandaries. Further, the respondents to the survey noted that the principle of respect for autonomy may conflict in some instances with the principle of beneficence or the principle of justice.

At the level of rules derived from the principles, the medical geneticists noted the general rule of respecting clients' freedom to make their own decisions or preserving the confidentiality of information about clients may need to be qualified, or even breached, in light of other weighty considerations. These limits may be set by the counselors' own moral convictions, as in the case of prenatal diagnosis for sex selection, or by substantial harms that are likely to occur to third parties—for example, if the members of an extended family are not informed about a diagnosis of Huntington's disease or if a husband is told that he is not the biological father of a genetically afflicted child born to his wife.

A second conclusion that can be drawn from geneticists' responses to these three clinical cases is that U.S. geneticists, as a group, are more likely to give higher priority to the principle of respect for autonomy than are geneticists from other nations. This tendency was most pronounced in the sex selection case but was present, as well, in the greater willingness of non-U.S. geneticists to breach confidentiality in the Huntington's disease case. Only in the third case, which involved nonpaternity, were non-U.S. geneticists slightly more likely to cite autonomy-based reasons than were U.S. geneticists.

Possible Future Challenges to the Predominant View

In the concluding part of this chapter, I will attempt to extrapolate from current situations in genetic counseling or health policy to imagine what types of situations may confront genetic counselors in the future. In the extrapolation I will present three scenarios about possible futures. Each scenario is slightly more global and more policy oriented than the preceding.

Scenario 1

In vitro fertilization (IVF) clinics are offering a diversified battery of diagnostic tests for preimplantation embryos. Not only can the early embryos be tested for common genetic and chromosomal disorders, like the trisomies, Duchenne's muscular dystrophy, and cystic fibrosis. The preimplantation tests can also detect predispositions to such problems as early coronary artery disease, a tendency toward low-normal stature, and a slight tendency toward obesity.

Genetic counseling clinics begin to be asked to run the same battery of tests during the first trimester of pregnancy after chorionic villus sampling (CVS). How do you respond to clients who make this request? Why?

This scenario extrapolates from the increasing use of preimplantation diagnosis by IVF clinics, the sex-selection case discussed above, and the probable successes of the worldwide Human Genome Project. It illustrates potential problems associated with the traditional emphasis of genetic counselors on respecting clients' freedom to make their own decisions.

As in the case of prenatal diagnosis for sex selection, this scenario raises the question of counselors or clinics setting moral limits on the types of services they are willing to provide. The autonomy-based rights of clients to secure information about a developing fetus may in some cases collide with the freedom of genetic counselors and clinics to focus their attention on serious medical problems that are diagnosable prenatally. However, there is a difference in this scenario between two ways of respecting autonomy. It would seem that the genetic counselor could respect the autonomy of the would-be clients only through positive action, that is, by performing the prenatal diagnosis requested. In contrast, the clients could respect the autonomy of reluctant or unwilling genetic counselors simply by forbearing, that is, by not pressing their request for prenatal diagnosis of cosmetic conditions.

This scenario implicitly raises questions about possible limits of the beneficence-based duty to prevent harm to a future child. There is in the request for prenatal diagnosis to detect a tendency toward low-normal stature more than a hint of perfectionism in the prospective parents. This tendency to perfectionism, when combined with questionable metaphysical assumptions about the interchangeability of fetuses, can lead to a seemingly endless quest for the ideal child (Rothman 1987). The metaphor that comes to mind is that of a potter trying to make a perfect vase. If a minor flaw is detected, or if the vessel becomes a bit lopsided in the molding process, the clay is simply removed from the wheel, broken down, and the potter starts anew. In my view, prospective parents who seek perfection in their children will be sadly disappointed—by the teenage years if not before!

This first scenario also illustrates potential conflicts between the autonomy of prospective fathers and the autonomy of prospective mothers. There is a clear differential between the two parties, in terms of physical and emotional harm, when one considers the possibility of repeated cycles of early pregnancy, prenatal diagnosis, and selective abortion. Genetic counselors may have an important role to play in protecting pregnant women from the overweening demands of biological fathers.

Scenario 2

> The Minnesota Health Insurance Plan (MHIP), modeled on a similar plan in Ontario, Canada, provides a basic level of health care for every resident in the state who chooses to join the plan. One requirement for participation in the plan is that every member must undergo a battery of tests for genetic traits, conditions, and susceptibilities, which then become a permanent part of his or her medical record. These tests are applied to consenting newcomers to the state when they establish residency and to infants, with parental consent, at the time of birth. There are no prenatal tests required as a condition for participation.
>
> The test results for adults are discussed with them alone. Minors' test results are discussed only with their parents. The primary rationale for the program is that it allows for early intervention to prevent or ameliorate serious or life-threatening conditions. In addition, the program is likely to help contain costs. Health economists have estimated that the genetic screening plan will produce a net benefit of $25 million per year for the state, if 75% of eligible residents participate. No one can be excluded from MHIP on the basis of test results.
>
> Do you consider such a genetic-testing requirement in a state-sponsored health insurance plan to be morally justifiable? Why or why not?

This scenario extrapolates from current neonatal screening programs, provincial health insurance plans in provinces such as Ontario, Canada, the Oregon health insurance plan for Medicaid recipients, and the underwriting practices of some U.S. life insurance and health insurance companies. It assumes that a progressive state like Minnesota will pioneer in planning and implementing state-based comprehensive health insurance plans for their residents.

A first point to be noted about this scenario is a subtlety in the distinction between voluntary and mandatory programs. MHIP is, in name and in fact, a voluntary program. Yet this state-sponsored health insurance plan may be so attractive, in comparison with privately offered plans, that residents of Minnesota conclude that they have no real choice in the matter. In the past when residents of Ontario were charged a monthly premium, some residents asserted, "since it costs only [x] dollars per month I can't afford not to belong."

This scenario also makes clear the potential benefits of genetic testing and screening for the individuals tested, given the proper set of social conditions. Nothing is said in the scenario about the availability of gene therapy. All that is required for benefit to the people tested is that conditions, traits, or susceptibilities be detectable for which early intervention is possible as a preventive measure. The benefits that accrue to individuals as improvements in their health status also translate into cost savings for the state government that sponsors the program.

Equally striking in this scenario is the method by which the stigmatization or discrimination often associated with genetic screening programs is avoided. The most important guarantee in MHIP is that the results of genetic testing cannot be used to exclude anyone from participation in the health insurance plan. Thus, the concern about what is viewed as unjust discrimination on the basis of one's genes (which one did not, in any case, choose) is effectively neutralized. The protection of individual privacy in the scenario is limited; that is, the results of genetic testing are included in the medical record, to which many people may have access. Yet even this sacrifice of the autonomy-based right to privacy may be considered worthwhile, if the costs of a program are reasonable and if the program provides guarantees against exclusion on the basis of test results.

A final lesson from this scenario is that a pioneering health insurance program developed by one progressive state may not be sufficient to alleviate people's concerns about stigmatization or unjust discrimination. For example, members of MHIP would be well provided with essential health care services as long as they resided in the state of Minnesota, but if they moved to another state without such a program, they might in fact be worse off as former MHIP members than as non-participants. In the new state former MHIP members might find that test results contained in their Minnesota medical records complicated the purchase of private health insurance—or even made it impossible. Further, even within Minnesota the question would surely arise whether private life insurance underwriters could have access to genetic test results compiled by MHIP.

Thus, regional or even national programs or standards will need to be in place if state-sponsored programs are to succeed, and a solution in the health insurance sector may not automatically resolve problems faced by citizens in other spheres of their lives.

Scenario 3

The year is 2055, and a definitive genetic cure for the mutations that cause cystic fibrosis (CF) has recently been discovered, tested, and perfected. This target-specific mode of gene therapy takes a properly functioning gene to the site of the mutation, splices out and destroys the malfunctioning gene, and replaces it with the properly functioning gene. The new technique can be applied equally well to somatic and germ-line (sperm or egg) cells.

The World Health Organization (WHO) has recently announced a global program to eradicate all CF mutations from the human gene pool. The program is modeled on the earlier campaign to eliminate smallpox. All persons at risk will be required to undergo testing and, if found to be affected or heterozygous, to accept genetic treatment of both their somatic and reproductive cells. WHO estimates that the global campaign will succeed within 35 years, at the most, and that the effort, when completed, will save $40 billion annually (in 2050 dollars) in the world health budget.

In your view, would such a mandatory global campaign be morally justifiable? Why or why not?

This scenario is extrapolated from past and present programs aimed at controlling serious infectious diseases. These programs include the worldwide campaign that eliminated smallpox, as well as state-based programs of mandatory immunization against such diseases as measles and polio.

A first question that can be raised about the proposed global program is whether it would properly be called a eugenics program. One's answer to this question depends on one's view regarding the essential features of such a program. The proposed program is certainly mandatory, as were earlier U.S. and German programs (Reilly 1991; Proctor 1988). Like the earlier programs, the proposed program is aimed at modifying the frequency of particular genes in populations. However, unlike the earlier programs, the proposed program seeks to eradicate a disease that is regarded as deleterious by all reasonable people and that is caused by clearly understood genetic mutations. Further, the WHO program would arguably be beneficial to everyone treated, including heterozygous carriers of a mutation that could cause CF in their offspring. Thus, the proposed program can be distinguished from earlier eugenics programs. If the term "eugenics" automatically implies moral reprehensibility, then this program is not eugenic. If the term "eugenics" is employed in a more descriptive and morally neutral manner, then the WHO program could be viewed as a morally justifiable eugenics program—that is, one aimed at eliminating a seriously deleterious gene from the human gene pool.

A second issue raised by this scenario is whether it is reasonable to draw an analogy between infectious disease and genetic disease. Proponents of the analogy point to the transmissibility of disease in both cases and argue that the mere direction or mode of transmission—horizontal or vertical—is less important than the spread of disease. Opponents of the analogy point out that while some infectious diseases are transmitted by intimate behavior, all genetic disease transmission occurs in the context of reproduction, one of the most intensely personal and private spheres of human life.

We are not told in Scenario 3 whether a voluntary program of genetic screening and gene therapy for CF has been tried and has failed. If it has not been tried, the burden of proof for the proponent of a mandatory program is heavier. Yet there may be plausible arguments, based on cost or the number of decades required to reach the goal, for the moral preferability of the mandatory approach in this case and all relevantly similar cases. If a voluntary program has been tried and has failed because of public inertia, a mandatory program might seem to be morally justifiable in this case, even to a civil libertarian, as a reasonable means to a highly desirable end.

Conclusion

I have noted that the traditional ethos of genetic counseling gives first priority to the principle of respect for autonomy. This principle is usually interpreted as requiring respect for clients' freedom in decision-making and the protection of confidential genetic information about clients. Several hard cases for genetic counselors have already indicated potential limits of the traditional ethos—in the United States and, even more decisively, abroad. Future advances in genetic science and technology may give rise to new situations in which the principle of respect for autonomy will be challenged, if not trumped, by other important ethical principles.

Acknowledgments

I thank the members of the Center for Biomedical Ethics at the University of Minnesota for their kind invitation to participate in a stimulating conference. I also appreciate the willingness of Dorothy Wertz and John Fletcher to share with me the cross-tabulations from their international survey, so that I could provide the reader with precise numbers of responses and the reasons given for those responses in my discussion of the case studies. My debt to colleagues in the National Reference Center for Bioethics Literature at the Kennedy Institute, who called my attention to relevant articles and books, is also great.

The research for this chapter was supported in part by Biomedical Research Support Grant RR-07136-18 from the National Institutes of Health.

Chapter 13

Neutrality Is Not Morality: The Ethics of Genetic Counseling

ARTHUR L. CAPLAN

The Ethos of Neutrality in Genetic Counseling

Those who do genetic counseling agree that it should always be done in a morally neutral manner. This is reflected in professional discussions of the goals of genetic counseling, in the norms that should govern the behavior of clinical geneticists and counselors, and in discussions of the techniques and methods that counselors should use to attain their goals. The long dominant view of the goals, norms, and methods thought appropriate in genetic counseling can be accurately described as an ethos of value neutrality (Antley 1979; Fraser 1974; President's Commission 1983b; World Medical Association 1987; Harris 1991; Rothman 1986).

Goals

The Code of Ethics recently promulgated by the National Society of Genetic Counselors (see Appendix B) provides a useful summary of the goals that professionals agree ought guide the process of counseling.

The goal of counseling is simple: The counselor is to empower the patient/client to make autonomous decisions. Autonomous decisions must be informed and free from coercion, but short of these ethical side-constraints, the values of the counselor should not play a role in setting the goals of clients.

The goal of simply providing information that the client can use to make a decision guided by their own values has been omnipresent

149

throughout the evolution of the specialty of clinical genetics in the United States over the past 20 years (Fraser 1974; Bosk 1985; Bosk, this volume). W. S. Sly in a classic article, "What is genetic counseling?," maintained the goal of counseling

> is the delivery of professional advice concerning the magnitude of, the implication of and the alternatives for dealing with the risk of occurrence of a hereditary disorder within a family. (Sly 1973)

The counselor is to provide accurate and understandable information. The responsibility for doing something with that information is not the counselor's, it is the client's (World Medical Association 1987; West 1988).

Norms

The norms of genetic counseling, as articulated in numerous books, articles, and codes of ethics, have—despite changes in the professional identity of those doing the counseling—remained relatively constant for the past 20 years. They exemplify the norm of value neutrality made famous by the fictional Sergeant Joe Friday on television's long-running detective series, *Dragnet*. Sergeant Friday, when called to the scene of a crime, would ask the victim to provide, "just the facts." Fridayism, the provision of the facts and only the facts, is entirely consistent with the textbook picture of the goals of genetic counseling, which sees the provision of purely factual information in the service of enhancing autonomous decision making by the client as the sole legitimate norm in the counseling process (Bosk this volume).

The presumption behind the norms guiding the actual conduct and methods of clinical genetics work is that autonomy, especially with respect to reproductive choices, can flourish only in a purely factual environment:

> clients are informed of all genetic risks, the methods available to refine the risks, the options available to deal with these risks, and the consequences likely to follow from each of the options. (Yarborough, Scott, and Dixon 1989)

A very influential article that appeared in the *American Journal of Human Genetics* discouraged the provision of anything other than the facts:

> This process [genetic counseling] involves . . . helping the individual or the family to (1) comprehend the medical facts . . . (2) appreciate the way in which heredity contributes to the disorder, (3) understand the options for dealing with risk of recurrence, (4) choose the course of action that seems

appropriate to them in view of their risk and their family goals. . . (5) make the best possible adjustment to the disorder. (Fraser 1974)

Methods

If the goal of counseling for the past 20 years has been to provide information to maximize client choices and the norm for doing so has been "Fridayism," the methods and techniques prescribed for achieving this goal while respecting this norm have, throughout this same period of time, been inhospitable to the overt appearance of professional values. Counseling has, for decades, been taught and depicted as an activity requiring moral neutrality concerning the actions, statements, and conduct of the counselor (Harris 1991; Bosk, this volume).

The commitment to moral neutrality concerning the counselor's behavior is best illustrated by the methodological recommendation that counseling be nondirective. It is the client's values and only the client's values that have any place in guiding decisions. Yarborough, Scott, and Dixon observe that the dominant view of genetic counseling insists that it be done,

> in a nondirective manner wherein the counselor maintains a morally neutral attitude about the particular choices clients may eventually make. (Yarborough et al. 1989)

Another clinical geneticist echoes this view when he writes,

> There is . . . general agreement that the doctor should respect the conscience and moral beliefs of the patient and not impose his personal moral values. (West 1988)

A stance favoring moral neutrality as the ethos of counseling was also noticeable in earlier writings on the subject. The distinguished clinical geneticist Robert Murray maintained in a 1974 article that genetic counseling

> is an educational process . . . but should not be directive in the decision-making process of the counselee. (Murray 1974)

Moral neutrality in counseling technique was prescribed in another widely cited paper:

> I judge it more advisable to give clients the genetic facts as objectively as possible and to refrain from giving the final recommendation of how these facts should be spliced into their personal equations. (Hsia 1979)

The ethos of value neutrality that dominates genetic counseling in America consists of three elements: the goal of maximizing patient or client choice, the norm of supplying only the facts, and the technique of nondirectiveness in the provision of information. Each of these elements has very little room for the expression of the values of the counselor.

The Distinctive Nature of the Ethos of Counseling

It is remarkable how the goals of enhancing patient autonomy, the technique of nondirectiveness, and the normative stance of absolute value neutrality differ from the goals, norms, and methods associated with other sorts of health care professional–patient encounters. Most areas of clinical medicine make no pretense of value neutrality.

If a test of a patient's blood lipid levels were to reveal a cholesterol count of 350, most doctors and public health experts would be astounded if this fact were merely reported to the patient with no prescriptive or normative recommendation. If a pediatrician were to examine a child and see a spine that displayed severe scoliosis and then give the parent of that child only a diagnosis with no recommendation for or against treatment, that physician certainly would not be praised by his or her peers for respecting the autonomous decision-making authority of the parent. The failure to offer a prescriptive recommendation concerning treatment would probably be seen as grounds for a malpractice charge due to culpable negligence.

Suppose a public health official or state child welfare official discovered an instance of child abuse or a failure to immunize a 10-year-old child against tetanus, polio, or diphtheria. They would hardly be expected to make client autonomy the central goal of their concern or to remain nondirective in counseling the parents of such children.

But this is not the ethos that prevails in the domain of clinical human genetics. Those doing counseling have been taught for more than 20 years that their goals, their norms, and their methods must be morally neutral. Counseling ought to aim at nothing more than the provision of facts about hereditary conditions and the options for choices available to the client in light of those facts. Counselors are taught (Marks, this volume) to provide facts about heredity without giving any hint as to their own values concerning the decision that a client ought to reach. It would be considered a gross violation of the ethos of counseling by most counselors for a counselor to criticize or disagree with the ultimate reproductive decision of a client.

The Challenge of the Genome Project to the Ethic of Neutrality

The question of whether moral neutrality is an adequate morality for clinical genetics and genetic counseling does not arise because those who do the counseling are ridden with self-doubt about the adequacy of the ethos that has dominated their work for more than two decades. It is not a result of ontological or epistemological challenges to the very possibility of value neutrality (Gervais, this volume). Nor is it provoked by complaints or disquiet on the part of clients, other health care providers, or the general public. Quite the opposite is true. Many experts in clinical genetics and counseling believe that it is the strict adherence to an ethos of value neutrality that has allowed the field to flourish.

My concern regarding the adequacy of the ethos of neutrality for counseling is rooted in the likelihood that those doing counseling will soon have a wealth of new information about the genetic makeup of eggs, sperm, embryos, fetuses, parents, and would-be parents as a result of ongoing efforts to map and sequence the human genome. If the genome project succeeds and a flood of new knowledge concerning the genetic contributions to human disease and disability becomes available, the ethos of moral neutrality will come under severe pressure for at least three reasons, the absence of enough adequately trained genetic counselors, uncertainty about what constitutes disease and health in the realm of genetics, and pressures to apply newly acquired genetic information in the service of containing the ever-escalating cost of health care (Caplan 1992a).

Who Will Act as Counselors?

One direct result of a quantum increase in information about the human genome is that the existing number of professionals available to provide counsel to those who seek access to this information will be completely and utterly inadequate. If the number of people seeking testing and counseling were to merely triple or quadruple there would not be enough clinical geneticists and genetic counselors around to handle them. Even if the numbers of counseling programs were to double or triple, the demand with person-hours for mass screening and counseling programs would quickly overwhelm the genetic counseling profession. Inevitably, the task of counseling will revert to primary care physicians, nurses, social workers, and other front-line health care professionals. These are groups, however, who have little formal training in genetics (Harris 1991), who rarely adhere to an ethos of value neutrality in their interactions with patients, and who are not likely to warm to suggestions that they need to suddenly adopt such an ethos when the conversation turns to heredity. Nor are their patients likely to accept the imposition of a special ethic regarding genetic information that allows only the person doing the counseling to provide facts and insists that they be nondirective when such an ethos does not prevail in other aspects of their relationships with providers.

Pressure on the ethos of neutrality will grow in proportion to the increase in what is known about variations in the human genome flowing from the Human Genome Project. The expansion of knowledge concerning the genetic basis of human phenotypes will raise obvious questions about what states, both mental and physical, constitute or are linked with health, disease, impairment, normality, and abnormality.

Uncertainty about the Meaning of New Genetic Knowledge

The field of clinical genetics has been confined until relatively recently to the detection of and counseling about highly unusual, uncommon, and often devastating genetic anomalies. The detection of extra or missing chromosomes, structural chromosomal abnormalities, or inborn errors of metabolism, although not simple, has, nevertheless, as its goal the detection of clear cut biological anomalies. The majority of these anomalies result, given certain developmental and environmental circumstances, in readily detectable phenotypic conditions, states, or symptoms. The consequences of most of the genetic conditions now at the center of genetic counseling are incapacitating, life-threatening, or both. One does not have to engage in elaborate arguments about the value of life or the quality of life to acknowledge that there are deleterious effects associated with Hurler disease, trisomy 13, Lesch–Nyhan syndrome, or PKU disease for those possessing these genetic constitutions (West 1988). Although there are many grounds for disagreement about whether efforts ought be made to screen or test for these conditions and what should be done if they are found to exist, there is little room for dispute as to the disvalued phenotypic consequences associated with these genomic states.

While most agree that anencephaly, spina bifida, Tay–Sachs disease, or trisomy 18 are to be disvalued because they are associated with impairment, dysfunction, or premature death, the prospect for obtaining agreement about the meaning, significance, and disease status of soon-to-be discovered genetic differences among human beings is far from clear. Simply finding polymorphisms at the genome level (e.g., within genes coding for blood types or skin colors) can be viewed as having little or great import depending on how such discoveries are presented and understood. For some prospective parents telling them that their fetus is "different" or that they are carriers of "unusual" genotypes may be enough to affect their reproductive behavior.

The genetic contribution to many common diseases and disorders whose disvalued status is not in dispute (i.e., cancer, Alzheimer disease, severe depression) will be made clearer as scientific understanding of the structure and composition of the genome increases. But more will also be learned about the genetic basis of other conditions (i.e., allergies, phobias, anxiety, short stature, poor dexterity, poor complexion) where there are fewer obvious points of agreement as to whether or not they should be disvalued much less classified as diseases or impairments.

The genome project is also likely to reveal a good deal of structural and anatomic information about variation among genomes for which there will be no clear understanding of the function of variation. Greater knowledge of structure without a corresponding knowledge of function provides ample opportunities for confusion, dispute, and disagreement about the significance of this information for determinations of the health or diseased state of those persons or groups who possess different or rare genomes. An ethics of neutrality is not likely to be as serviceable when the "facts" about heredity are much more controversial than they have been for most of the history of genetic counseling (Burke and Kolker 1991; Caplan 1992a, 1992b).

Cost Containment and Counseling

The ethos of neutrality with respect to counseling will also be challenged by the impact new knowledge resulting from the genome project will have in the arena of health policy. There is every reason to presume that the costs of health care will continue to increase well into the first few decades of the next century (Callahan 1987). Many experts (Callahan 1987; Churchill 1987; Menzel 1990) are convinced that the explicit rationing of access to health care as a matter of public policy is the only solution to controlling the high costs associated with modern health care.

If it is possible to reduce the cost of care by preventing the birth or compelling the early treatment of those likely to have costly diseases and disorders, then the ethos of neutrality dominant today with respect to both goals and conduct in genetic counseling will be fiercely challenged. Many will see the application of new knowledge concerning the genome as a legitimate and ethical way for society to decrease the burden of paying the costs associated with disease, disorder, and dysfunction (Holmes 1991). Historically, new information about the genetic basis of behavior has led to powerful movements in American public policy for the utilization of that information for the good of society (Reilly 1991).

Political pressure for genetic counselors to take a normative stance, which accommodates society's need to decrease the cost of diseases and disorders with strong hereditary origins, will escalate as more becomes known about the role played by heredity in human health. Public health will incorporate more and more information about the hereditary basis of disease into its increasingly proactive and prophylactic stance toward the goal of disease prevention. It will become increasingly difficult to remain value neutral if the information supplied by the genome project permits cost savings through 'prudent' or 'responsible' reproductive choices (Blumberg 1987).

If Genetic Counseling Is Nondirective Is It Morally Neutral?

How inhospitable to the impending assault on value neutrality will genetic counseling be? Is the ethos of neutrality likely to yield as the work of the genome project proceeds in the United States and other nations and the knowledge base for testing, screening, and counseling grows? If, despite the oft professed allegiance to an ethos of neutrality, genetic counseling is not and has not ever really been conducted in accordance with that ethos, then the absorption of new genetic knowledge into counseling may meet with less resistance then might be expected.

While those who teach and write about counseling depict the goals, norms, and methods used in morally neutral terms, there are many reasons to think they are simply kidding themselves as to the moral content of their actual work. The few studies that have been done of the content of genetic counseling and of the attitudes of genetic counselors reveal wide variations in their beliefs and practices (Bosk, this volume; LeRoy, this volume; Sorenson, Kavanaugh, and Mucatel 1981; Rothman 1986; Wertz and Fletcher 1989, 1990). In practice, an ethos of neutrality exists alongside a wide spectrum of beliefs, attitudes, and conduct. These differences suggest that value neutrality is hardly the order of the day in genetic counseling. When differences in the ability of professionals and clients to understand and process probabilistic information are weighed into the assessment of value neutrality (Lappé this volume), it becomes even harder to believe that a single style of presenting information is or could be consistent with a desire to remain value neutral.

Could genetic counseling be morally neutral? What would it look like if it was? The only way to answer this question is to clarify what might be meant by prescriptions requiring that counseling be morally neutral.

One of the reasons why it is possible to argue that genetic counseling is not morally neutral is that it is not exactly obvious, despite the frequency with which such claims are made, what an ethos of neutrality entails. The most frequent injunctions as to how to achieve an ethos of neutrality are exemplified in warnings that counseling must be nondirective. Moral neutrality is often equated with nondirectiveness (Yarborough, Scott, and Dixon 1989; West 1988; Harris 1991).

Of all of the possible ways in which counseling might be seen as value neutral, nondirectiveness seems to have been of the greatest historical importance to professionals who have written about the ethics of this activity. Yet, oddly, the issue of directiveness does not seem to have anything to do with avoiding or eliminating a specific set of norms, values, or principles. Rather, nondirectiveness is used to describe the stance that the counselor should adopt toward the counselee, one of openness and a willingness to listen. Nondirectiveness has its roots in a theoretical position within psychiatry, social work, and psychoanalysis that prescribes nondirectiveness as the best stance for eliciting information from a patient so that the patient may come to have insight about his or her psychological problems.

Directive counseling would permit or require the counselor to be active, willing to engage in challenge, argument, and confrontation with clients. Those who favor nondirective counseling among genetic counseling professionals are usually referring not to a neutral or indifferent moral outlook but, rather, to a passive role in which counselors try to be responsive to client needs and questions and avoid challenges or confrontations in seeking to accomplish their educational goals (Antley 1979)

Seen in this light it quickly becomes obvious that the discussions of the appropriateness of 'directedness' with respect to genetic counseling have little to do with ethics or values. Those who insist on nondirective counseling (Marks, this volume; Fine, this volume; Lappé, this volume) do so because they believe that counselors will be most effective at communicating and conveying information if they listen carefully to those who seek their help and avoid directly challenging or confronting their clients. But, the effectiveness of nondirectiveness as a technique, or the best technique, for ascertaining client needs and conveying information is amenable to empirical assessment. It is simply a mistake to equate nondirectiveness in counseling with value neutrality. Nondirective counseling need not presuppose any particular moral outlook but it is quite compatible with many prescriptive stances.

Admittedly, there are moral constraints over the kinds of techniques that are permissible to use in the context of a counseling session be it directive or not (i.e., no coercion, no hectoring, no threats, no rudeness, etc.). But imposing these sorts of constraints over the process of counseling is surely not to advocate adhering to an ethic of moral neutrality.

Passivity and responsiveness may be preferable to aggression and proactivity in trying to talk about genetic information (or anything else for that matter!). But those who insist on the desirability of nondirective counseling are doing so on grounds that have little to do with morality but rather a lot to do with their beliefs concerning what is and is not effective in facilitating communication. The limits on what counselors can do and how they ought behave are set by beliefs about what allows successful communication, they do not redefine the adoption of a value-neutral ethic for genetic counseling.

Whatever else is meant by those who recommend counseling only proceed with a value-neutral morality, the assessment of the importance of nondirectiveness does not hinge on a moral argument. The value of nondirectiveness keys on the answer to the question as to which psycho-social techniques are most effective in ensuring communication between counselor and counselee. The question of how directive to be must be settled by empirical inquiries into what techniques actually do produce the most success with respect to the successful communication of information about heredity. Decisions about the desirability of directiveness do not require a value neutral ethics. They do require empirical evidence about the impact of counseling, evidence that seems to be in precious short supply because the need for it has been obscured by its connection with ethical matters.

The other important reason evident in the literature of clinical genetics from the past two decades for an ethic of value neutrality for genetic counseling is to prohibit counselors from making particular recommendations or prescribing specific courses of action to their clients. The insistence on nonprescriptiveness in counseling has its roots in the history of the goals that have fueled clinical genetics (Kessler 1980).

When genetic counseling first appeared it was clearly, explicitly, and unabashedly linked to achieving eugenic goals. At the turn of the century and for roughly the next three decades, health care professionals sought to make genetic counseling available to persons in the hope that they would discourage those likely to have impaired, diseased, or mentally defective children from having them. Some also hoped to encouraging those whom they saw as having positive genetic endowments to have lots of children (Kessler 1980; Hubbard 1986). As the scientific underpinnings for both negative and positive eugenics came under challenge in the 1940s and 1950s, and as the horrors of social policies built on race hygiene in Nazi Germany were revealed (Proctor 1988, Reilly 1991), the emphasis shifted from eugenic goals to the goals of prevention.

The eugenic origins of genetic counseling lingered on in the United States in the 1960s and early 1970s, not so much in clinical genetics but in mass screening programs which had a more public health orientation (Hubbard 1986). The goal of prevention loomed large in the numerous mass screening programs that were instituted in the name of public health. Programs to screen for sickle cell disease, PKU, Tay–Sachs, and Down syndrome were all instituted in the hopes that persons at risk of having children with these diseases would receive counseling that would stress the importance of prevention—meaning either refraining from procreation or choosing sterilization or abortion.

Obviously, genetic screening and counseling that has prevention as its goal is not morally neutral (Rothman 1986). Those working in mass screening programs in the 1960s and 1970s were to identify certain states as desirable and others as undesirable and were expected to counsel in light of the risks of creating undesirable outcomes.

Eugenic goals have not completely disappeared from the realm of genetic testing and counseling. When the Prime Minister of Singapore decided a few years ago to offer cash incentives to families with high IQs to have more children, when various provinces in the Peoples' Republic of China adopt sterilization policies for the mentally ill and retarded, when persons who have conceived a child with 47,XYY syndrome are advised to abort the pregnancy, or when a sperm bank operates in California with the explicit goal of creating smart children who can lead future generations, genetic information is being used in the light of certain values to guide reproduction (Chadwick 1987). When the state of California offers maternal serum α-fetoprotein screening to all pregnant women it does so in the hope that some of those who are found to have children with neural tube defects will choose not to bring them to term; thereby, preventing the state from having to bear the burden of their care. The ethos behind prevention is neither nondirective nor nonprescriptive. This does not make it wrong, but it would be incorrect to say it is consistent with an ethos of neutrality.

In the late 1970s and 1980s some in the profession of genetic counseling began to become uncomfortable with the goal of prevention. The most obvious reason for this discomfort was that the only realistic means of prevention for most genetic diseases detected *in utero* was abortion. One way for coping with the controversial nature of abortion was for the genetic counseling to shift away from prescribing prevention toward a more value neutral ethic that emphasized the need to respect client autonomy. The shift from prevention toward an ethic that extols the virtue of enhancing client autonomy was reinforced by a general shift in the ethics of health care away from paternalism and beneficence toward an autonomy driven ethic in provider–patient relationships (Caplan 1992a).

What is not obvious, however, is that a shift away from an ethical stance favoring the prescription of eugenic or preventative goals toward one favoring respect for the autonomy of client decision making is in any way morally neutral. On the contrary, the shift toward an ethic that elevates client or patient autonomy above all other values is highly value laden and prescriptive.

Touting a nonprescriptive ethic is not the same thing as touting a morally neutral ethic. In reality those who believe genetic counseling should be both nonprescriptive and nondirective maintain these views because they believe that clients should have the final word over decisions and actions, and that they will be in a better position to make decisions if these norms are followed by counselors. This means that respect for autonomy and the desirability of informed, "rational" decision making are norms of critical importance. And this means that the ethic being taught, recommended, and defended is anything but morally neutral or value free (Yarborough, Scott, and Dixon 1989).

The advocacy of a morally neutral ethic by those in genetic counseling may be intended to avoid certain other problems. Sometimes those who advocate an ethic of moral neutrality warn against the counselor being judgmental toward clients. Moral neutrality is a way of indicating that counselors must be nonjudgmental about those they serve.

Similarly, an ethic of value neutrality is sometimes advanced as a way to warn against the covert smuggling of professional or personal counselor values into the counseling situation. It is intended to prohibit the utilization of tacit or covert values in the selection of information that is passed along to counselees.

Avoiding the use of covert values and advocating that counselors remain nonjudgmental may be sound strategies for effective genetic counseling. But they are also norms that are clearly motivated by the belief that the client's autonomy can be allowed to flourish only in certain environments. Respect for patient or client autonomy is clearly the ethic that underpins these sorts of recommendations.

Finally, the notion that genetic counseling must be morally neutral may be motivated by the concern that values not be allowed to influence or color the facts with respect to the presentation of information about the risks and consequences of particular genetic conditions or states. The facts must be given objectively (West 1988; Harris 1991).

One commonly hears counselors say that they feel obligated to present all the facts and all the options to their clients. Strictly adhering to the admonition to be morally neutral in the selection and transmission of information may lead counselors to simply dump information onto their clients. At its worst, informed consent in any area of health care can be treated as an exercise in truth dumping in which every fact, every option, every risk, and every benefit is unleashed on an unwitting and sometimes unwilling patient because the person giving the information feels that they must do so in a way that is completely value free. Such an exercise often leads to frustration rather than the enhancement of autonomy.

Since the ethic of genetic counseling is surely committed to autonomy enhancement, the idea that information is value free or can be presented in a value free manner makes little sense. Surely the counselor must exercise some judgment over what information to present and how to best present it. Trying to preserve the objectivity of information about heredity by insisting on the value free nature of counseling leads to information overload—not informed decision making.

Why Has an Ethic of Moral Neutrality Dominated Genetic Counseling for the Past Twenty Years?

Why has a distinctive ethos of moral neutrality dominated genetic counseling in the United States and other Western nations for the past two decades? Abuse carried out under the banner of eugenics and the controversy over elective abortion are key reasons.

Those who established the field of clinical genetics in the years after WW II were keenly aware of the tie that existed between genetics and the Holocaust. They also knew that there were powerful strains of racism and bigotry in evidence in the field of genetics in the United States, Canada, the United Kingdom, and other countries in the prewar years (Kessler 1980). The emphasis on moral neutrality as the guiding ethic of clinical genetics was a reaction against the utilization of genetics and clinical genetics in the service of an ideology that led to mass genocide in Germany (Proctor 1988) and coercive sterilization in the United States and other nations (Reilly 1991).

Few areas of science have had to live with the historical legacy of abuse that haunts clinical genetics. The history of the twentieth century ends all arguments about whether or not it is possible to abuse genetic information. As a result, few areas of science or medicine have been so keen to restrict or confine the role played by professionals to matters of fact, not value as genetic counseling.

The other major reason for the emergence of an ethic of value neutrality in genetic counseling is the link between counseling and reproduction. In America, genetic counseling came of age at the same time as a political movement to carve out a fundamental right to privacy with respect to reproduction regarding contraception, abortion, and sexual conduct was emerging. The right of a woman to choose whether or not to bear a child emerged in the late 1960s and early 1970s. At the time this right was being articulated, a shift was taking place in the composition of those doing genetic counseling from M.D.s to M.A.s and from men to women (Burke and Kolker 1991; Bosk, this volume). The women who began to dominate the counseling field were hardly unaware of the importance of reproductive rights for women and the controversy over the right to abortion on demand. The right to privacy meant that women had to remain free to choose whether or not they would have a child regardless of what genetic testing revealed. The fragility of that right could not have been lost on the women who were beginning to dominate the field of genetic counseling.

Not only did genetic counseling emerge in tandem with the right to reproductive privacy, it was inextricably intertwined with the issue of abortion. The only option available to women or parents in almost all situations where congenital anomalies were discovered prenatally was abortion. Abortion was and remains a subject that generates enormous moral conflict. An ethic of value neutrality provided some space for clinical genetics from the abortion controversy. Genetic counselors could not be accused of favoring or promoting abortion if they adhered to a strict ethic of value neutrality.

The Time Has Come to Abandon the Ethic of Neutrality

Are there sufficient reasons to abandon the ideal of moral neutrality in genetic counseling and attempt to initiate a debate about what ethos should be put in its place? This question is especially acute when the focus of moral discussion shifts from the clinical to that of public health policy. The danger of misunderstanding and misapplication of the information likely to be created by the Human Genome Project suggests that the time has come to abandon the pretense of moral neutrality, both in the clinical setting and in the public policy arena.

Clinical Practice

The avowal of an ethic of neutrality probably did provide room for clinical genetics to grow despite the long shadow cast by Nazi eugenics. The ethic of neutrality was indisputably helpful in providing a buffer for the field from the heated controversy over the right of women to elect abortions.

But promoting value neutrality as the moral ideal for counselors no longer makes sense. The abuses of the Nazi era no longer threaten the existence of the field. And an ethic of neutrality is unlikely to provide much cover from the current divisive debates about abortion in which you are either seen as for or against it. Moreover, the flood of new information soon to sweep into clinical genetics from the findings of the Human Genome Project raises many other questions about the aims and goals of clinical genetics that go beyond the question of the morality of elective abortion.

Value neutrality is no longer healthy for the practice of clinical genetics. It deflects attention away from the question of whether neutrality actually prevails in counseling sessions and, if it does, what counselors and clients think it actually means. The relative paucity of studies of the actual practices of genetic counselors is partly a result of the dominance of the value neutral ethos among those in the field.

Value neutrality discourages those in the field from coming to grips with the central ethical question that now confronts the field—how to define genetic disease and disorder in order to lay out appropriate targets for testing and counseling. When the genetic abnormalities, which were the object of testing and counseling, were relatively noncontroversial in terms of their dysfunctional and disvalued status, the definition of genetic disease could be put aside. As more and more information becomes available on more and more genetic conditions this question can no longer be avoided. Ducking the question of what it is that clinical genetics seeks to detect and possibly treat has led many persons with disabilities to distrust the motives and goals of those in clinical genetics (Blumberg 1987).

With a mountain of new information about the human genome looming in the not so distant future, genetic counseling can no longer afford to ignore the question of what sorts of disorders and diseases it wishes to discover, why, and what exactly it wants to say about them. Definitions of genetic disease and disorder must be spelled out so that they are available for criticism and challenge by clients as well as by those inside and outside the field.

An ethos of value neutrality also makes it very difficult for patients to hold counselors accountable for their conduct. If neutrality is the avowed ethos but no clear consensus exists as to what the ethos involves in terms of actual behavior and conduct, then it will be difficult for clients to know when and if a counselor is deviating from neutrality in the provision of information. If any and all behavior is compatible with an avowed stance of value neutrality then the ability to ensure quality in genetic counseling is severely impaired.

Value neutrality also leaves counselors powerless in the face of what may be immoral requests on the part of clients. If families come seeking testing and counseling so that they can indulge their taste for a child of a particular sex, or if, for some personal reasons, they want a child with a particular disease or handicap (Nance, this volume), or because they hope to create a tissue donor (Kearney and Caplan 1992), the counselor bound by strict value neutrality can say nothing. As the range of traits and conditions correlated with genetic states begins to grow, the requests of parents are likely to grow as well. At some point parents are likely to begin making requests for testing and counseling that clearly fall in the realm of genetic improvement and enhancement rather than in the domain of dysfunction and disease. An ethic of value neutrality provides no foundation for counselors to try and dissuade parents from making choices that are frivolous, silly, or malicious.

Public Health and Public Policy

Failure to shift away from an ethic of value neutrality not only restricts what can be said and done in the clinical setting it may disenfranchise those providing genetic counseling and testing from participation in the determination of public policy, with respect to genetics and the use of the new knowledge arising from the genome project. For example, will genetic counselors remain silent in the face of questions as to whether or not the government or the general public has a legitimate stake in the quantity and quality of children that are born? Since Americans accept the idea that the government ought to try and improve the health of children by means of prenatal care and family planning programs will they not insist that new genetic knowledge be used to improve the health and welfare of children? And if the state has a legitimate interest in minimizing the burden illness imposes on those who pay taxes, it may be that the state will take a far more involved and even coercive stance toward influencing reproductive decisions. If other nations choose to pursue explicitly eugenic goals in their public policies concerning reproduction (Chadwick 1987) what will be the basis for disagreement or criticism if only a value-neutral ethic is available to those in the field of clinical genetics?

Value neutrality leaves those who do genetic counseling in no position to participate in debates about what priorities ought to be set on research in the realm of genetics. The question of how to allocate dollars among testing, screening, counseling, public education, therapy, and rehabilitation is one that surely demands that the views of the genetic counseling community be heard. But despite the explosion of new information resulting from success in mapping and sequencing more and more areas of the human genome, a value-neutral stance is not the best way to try to influence how money ought to be spent in light of this new information.

Setting out value neutrality as a moral ideal also leaves the door open to others who might not have the same moral scruples to counsel or offer their services. The fact that an explicitly and proudly eugenicist sperm bank, the Repository for Germinal Choice, has been operating in Southern California for many years indicates that there are other segments of society who will want to use new genetic information to serve their particular vision of what the future genetic makeup of the human species ought to be. Value neutrality will work as an ethic only if there are no other competing groups offering prescriptively based counseling.

Lastly, a stance of value neutrality may foster a sense of irresponsibility about reproduction and genetics. If reproductive choice is simply a matter of individual choice and nothing more, if no moral argument or persuasion is considered licit, then the message the profession is sending to its clients and the public is that you can do with your gametes as you please. It may be true that we ought not allow government to take a strong hand in legislating who can and cannot reproduce (although this is hardly a value neutral position!). But there is a big difference between not wanting to become involved in legislative and judicial matters pertaining to the use of genetic information in making reproductive choices and not having anything to say about the rights, duties, and responsibilities of those who choose to reproduce.

Ethics is not the same as the law. It is possible to believe that something is morally wrong and yet not believe it should be outlawed. Similarly, it is possible to believe that an act or policy is morally right or good without believing that there is a role for the state, the courts, or the legislature.

If those in genetic counseling still believe that the lessons of history indicate that a gap must be allowed to exist between the practice of clinical genetics and public policy, this does not mean that the only way to ensure that that gap exists is to cling to an ethos of value neutrality. Ironically, to do so is to leave the field to others who will not necessarily be so like-minded.

There are many who will see the influx of new information from the Human Genome Project as providing an opportunity to advance their social, ideological, racial, or economic goals. Value neutrality, whether possible or not in the clinical setting, is simply not an adequate ethic in the public policy arena. It is precisely the information sought by those involved in the genome project that points toward the inadequacies of the current ethic in genetic counseling.

PART IV

Appendix

Appendix A

National Society of Genetic Counselors Code of Ethics

Preamble

Genetic counselors are health professionals with specialized education, training, and experience in medical genetics and counseling

The National Society of Genetic Counselors (NSGC) is an organization that furthers the professional interests of genetic counselors, promotes a network for communication within the profession, and deals with issues relevant to human genetics.

With the establishment of this code of ethics the NSGC affirms the ethical responsibilities of its members and provides them with guidance in their relationships with self, clients, colleagues, and society. NSGC members are expected to be aware of the ethical implications of their professional actions and to adhere to the guidelines and principles set forth in this code.

Introduction

A code of ethics is a document which attempts to clarify and guide the conduct of a professional so that the goals and values of the profession might best be served. The NSGC Code of Ethics is based upon relationships. The relationships outlined in this code describe who genetic counselors are for themselves, their clients, their colleagues, and society. Each major section of this code begins with an explanation of one of these relationships, along with some of its values and characteristics. Although certain values are found in more than one relationship, these common values result in different guidelines within each relationship.

No set of guidelines can provide all the assistance needed in every situation, especially when different relationships appear to conflict. Therefore, when considered appropriate for this code, specific guidelines for prioritizing the relationships have been stated. In other areas, some ambiguity remains, allowing for the experience of genetic counselors to provide the proper balance in responding to difficult situations.

Section I: Genetic Counselors Themselves

Genetic counselors value competence, integrity, dignity, and self-respect in themselves as well as in each other. Therefore, in order to be the best possible human resource to themselves, their clients, their colleagues, and society, genetic counselors strive to

1. Seek out and acquire all relevant information required for any given situation.
2. Continue their education and training.
3. Keep abreast of current standards of practice.
4. Recognize the limits of their own knowledge, expertise, and therefore competence in any given situation.
5. Be responsible for their own physical and emotional health as it impacts on their professional performance.

Section II: Genetic Counselors and Their Clients

The counselor-client relationship is based on values of care and respect for the client's autonomy, individuality, welfare, and freedom. The primary concern of genetic counselors is the interests of their clients. Therefore, genetic counselors strive to

1. Equally serve all who seek services.
2. Respect their client's beliefs, cultural traditions, inclinations, circumstances, and feelings.
3. Enable their clients to make informed independent decisions, free of coercion, by providing or illuminating the necessary facts and clarifying the alternatives and anticipated consequences.
4. Refer clients to other competent professionals when they are unable to support the clients.
5. Maintain as confidential any information received from clients, unless released by the client.
6. Avoid the exploitation of their clients for personal advantage, profit, or interest.

Section III: Genetic Counselors and Their Colleagues

The genetic counselors' relationships with other genetic counselors, genetic counseling students, and health professionals are based on mutual respect, caring, cooperation, support, and a shared loyalty to their professions and goals. Therefore, genetic counselors strive to

1. Foster and protect their relationships with other genetic counselors and genetic counseling students by establishing mechanisms for peer support.
2. Encourage ethical behavior of colleagues.
3. Recognize the traditions, practices, and areas of competence of other health professionals and cooperate with them in providing the highest quality of service.
4. Work with their colleagues to reach consensus when issues arise about the role responsibilities of various team members so that clients receive the best possible services.

Section IV: Genetic Counselors and Society

The relationships of genetic counselors to society include interest and participation in activities that have the purpose of promoting the well-being of society. Therefore, genetic counselors strive to

1. Keep abreast of societal developments that may endanger the physical and psychological health of individuals.
2. Participate in activities necessary to bring about socially responsible change.
3. Serve as a source of reliable information and expert opinion for policy makers and public officials.
4. Keep the public informed and educated about the impact on society of new technological and scientific advances and the possible changes in society that may result from the application of these findings.
5. Prevent discrimination on the basis of race, sex, sexual orientation, age, religion, genetic status, or socioeconomic status.
6. Adhere to laws and regulations of society. However, when such laws are in conflict with the principles of the profession, genetic counselors work toward change that will benefit the public interest.

Acknowledgment

The above Appendix was reprinted with permission of the National Society of Genetic Counselors (NSGC) June, 1991, Human Sciences Press.

References

Ad Hoc Committee on Genetic Counseling of the American Society of Human Genetics. 1975. *American Journal of Human Genetics* 27:240–242.

American College of Physicians. 1989. "American College of Physicians Manual Part I: History; the Patient; Other Physicians." *Annals of Internal Medicine* 111:245–252.

American Society of Human Genetics. 1975. "Genetic Counseling." *American Journal of Human Genetics* 27:240–242.

Andrews, L. B. 1987. *Medical Genetics: A Legal Frontier.* Chicago: American Bar Foundation.

Annas, G. 1992. "The Human Genome Project as Social Policy: Implications for Clinical Medicine." *New York Academy of Medicine Bulletin* 68:126–134.

Antley, R. M. 1979. "The Genetic Counselor as Facilitator of the Counselee's Decision Process." Pp. 137–168 in *Genetic Counseling: Facts, Values and Norms,* edited by Capron, A. M., M. Lappé, R. F. Murray. New York: Alan R. Liss.

"Asymptomatic Infection with the AIDS Virus as a Handicap under the Rehabilitation Act of 1973." 1988. *Columbia Law Review* 88:563–586.

Austin, J. 1975. *How to Do Things with Words.* Cambridge: Harvard University Press.

Baker, D., J. Benkendorf, and A. Heimler. 1987. "Report from the Ad Hoc Committee on the Expanded Roles of Genetic Counselors." National Society of Genetic Counselors.

Beauchamp, T. L. and J. F. Childress. 1989. *Principles of Biomedical Ethics.* New York: Oxford University Press.

Becker, M. H. and I. Rosenstock. 1989. "Health Promotion, Disease Prevention, and Program Retention." Pp. 284–305 in *Handbook of Medical Sociology,* edited by Freeman, H. E., and S. Levine. Englewood Cliffs, NJ: Prentice Hall.

Beeson, D. and M. S. Golbus. 1985. "Decision Making: Whether or Not to Have Prenatal Diagnosis and Abortion for X-linked Conditions." *American Journal of Medical Genetics* 20:107–114.

Benkendorf, J. 1990. "Code of Ethics Update." *Perspectives of Genetic Counseling* 12:11.

Blakeslee, S. 1990. "Ethicists See Omen of an Era of Genetic Bias." *The New York Times*, December 27.

Blumberg, L. 1987. "Why Fetal Rights Must be Opposed." *Social Policy Journal* 18(2):40–41.

Bosk, C. L. 1992. *All God's Mistakes: Genetic Counseling in a Pediatric Hospital.* Chicago: University of Chicago Press.

Bosk, C. L. 1985. "The Fieldworker as Watcher and Witness." *Hastings Center Report* 15:10–14.

Brock, D. W. 1991. "The Ideal of Shared Decision Making Between Physicians and Patients." *Kennedy Institute of Ethics Journal* 1:28–47.

Brown, H. I. 1987. *Observation and Objectivity.* New York: Oxford University Press.

Bucher, R. and A. Strauss. 1961. "Professions in Process." *American Journal of Sociology Journal* 66(4):325–334.

Burke, M. and A. Kolker. 1991. "Counselor Risk Assessment and Directiveness in Prenatal Genetic Counseling." Paper presented at Annual Meeting of the Society for the Study of Social Problems, Cincinnati, OH.

Callahan, D. 1987. *Setting Limits.* New York: Simon and Schuster.

Caplan, A. L. 1992a. "If Gene Therapy is the Cure, What is the Disease?" Pp. 128–141 in *Gene Mapping: Using Law and Ethics as Guides*, edited by Annas, G. and S. Elias. New York: Oxford University Press.

Caplan, A. L. 1992b. *If I Were A Rich Man Could I Buy A Pancreas? And Other Essays on the Ethics of Health Care*, Bloomington, IN: Indiana University Press.

Capra, J. 1989. "Translating Genetics into English: The Public Education Experience." Pp. 121–125 in *Strategies in Genetic Counseling: Tools for Professional Advancement*, edited by Zellers, N. J. New York: Human Sciences Press.

Carter, C., K. Evans, J. A. Fraser-Roberts, and A. Buck. 1971. "Genetic Clinic: A Follow-up." *The Lancet* 1:281–285.

Chadwick, R. 1987. *Ethics, Reproduction and Genetic Control.* London: Routledge.

Chandler, K. 1990. "Senate Vote is First on Abortion Issue: Amended Bill Banning Medical Use of Fetuses is Tabled." *Star Tribune*, Section B:5.

Churchill, L. 1987. *Rationing Health Care in America.* Notre Dame: Notre Dame University Press.

Clifford, K. A. and R. P. Luculano. 1987. "AIDS and Insurance: The Rationale for AIDS-Related Testing." *Harvard Law Review* 100:1806–1825.

Collins, D. L. and R. N. Schimke. 1988. "Innovations in Human Genetics Education: College Course Work in Human Genetics for Elementary, Middle, and High School Educators in Kansas." *American Journal of Human Genetics* 42:633–634.

Copeland, K. 1989. "Can Nondirectiveness be Non-helpful?" *Perspectives in Genetic Counseling* 11:3.

Corsini, R. J. 1979. *Current Psychotherapies.* Itasca, Illinois: F. E. Peacock Publishers.

de Fiebre, C. 1991. "DNA Testing Questioned Anew after Lab Opening." *Star Tribune*, Section B:1.

Department of Health, Education and Welfare. "Grant 5 D02AH01027 and 5 D12AH00792."

Dumars, K., J. Burns, S. Kessler, J. Marks, and A. P. Walker. "Genetic Associates: Their Training Role and Function." In A Conference Report, 1979, Washington, DC, U. S. Department of Health, Education and Welfare.

Elkins, T. E., T. G. Stoval, S. Wilroy, and J. V. Dacus. 1986. "Attitudes of Mothers of Children with Down Syndrome Concerning Amniocentesis, Abortion and Prenatal Genetic Counseling Techniques." *Obstetrics and Gynecology* 68:181–184.

"Employment Discrimination Implications of Genetic Screening in the Workplace." 1983. *Title VII and the Rehabilitation Act* 10:323–347.

Engelhardt, H. T. 1986. *The Foundations of Bioethics.* New York: Oxford University Press.

Epstein, C. J. 1975. "Genetic Counseling: Present Status and Future Prospects." Pp. 110–128 in *Early Diagnosis and Prevention of Genetic Disease,* edited by Went, L. N., C. Vermeij-Keers, and A. G. van der Linden. Leiden: Leiden University Press.

Evans, M. I., S. F. Bottoms, and G. C. Critchfield. 1990. "Parental Perceptions of Genetic Risk: Correlation with Choice of Prenatal Diagnostic Procedures." *International Journal of Gynaecology and Obstetrics* 31:25–28.

Evers-Kiebooms, G. L. Denayer, and H. Van den Berghe. 1990. "A Child With Cystic Fibrosis: Subsequent Family Planning Decisions, Reproduction and Use of Prenatal Diagnosis." *Clinical Genetics* 37:207–215.

Feller, I. 1980. "Science and Technology in State and Local Governments Probems and Opportunites." Pp. 639–647 In *The Five-Year Outlook; Problems, Opportunities and Constraints in Science and Technology Vol. II.*

Fiatal, R. A. 1990. "DNA Testing and the Frye Standard." *FBI Law Enforcement Bulletin* 26–31.

Finley, W. H., S. C. Finley, and R. L. Dyer. 1987. "Survey of Medical Genetics Personnel." *American Journal of Human Genetics* 40:374–377.

Fletcher, J. C. 1988. *The Ethics of Genetic Control: Ending Reproductive Roulette.* New York: Prometheus Books.

Fletcher, J. C. and D. C. Wertz. 1987. "Ethical Aspects of Prenatal Diagnosis: Views of U. S. Medical Genetics." *Clinical Perinatology* 14:293–312.

Fletcher, J. C. and D. C. Wertz 1987. "Ethics and Human Genetics: A Cross-Cultural Perspective." *Seminars in Perinatology* 11:224–228.

Fox, R. C. and J. Swazey. 1974. *The Courage to Fail: A Social View of Organ Transplants and Dialyses.* Chicago: University of Chicago Press.

Fraser, F. C. 1974. "Genetic Counseling." *American Journal of Human Genetics* 26:636–659.

Fraser, F. C. 1979. "Introduction: The Development of Genetic Counseling." Pp. 5–15 in *Genetic Counseling: Facts, Values and Norms,* edited by Capron, A. M., M. Lappé, R. F. Murray. New York: Alan R. Liss.

Freidson, E. 1970. *Profession of Medicine.* New York: Dodd, Mead & Co.

Frets, F. and M. Niermeyer. 1990. "Reproductive Planning after Genetic Counseling: A Perspective from the Past Decade." *Clinical Genetics* 38:295–306.

Frets, P. G., H. J. Duivenvoorden, and F. Berhage. 1990b. "Factors Influencing the Reproductive Decision After Genetic Counseling." *American Journal of Medical Genetics* 35:496–502.

Frets, P. G., H. J. Duivenvoorden, and F. Berhage. 1990. "Model Identifying the Reproductive Decision After Genetic Counseling." *American Journal of Medical Genetics* 35:503–509.

"Genetic Associates: Their Training Role and Function." in *A Conference Report,* edited by Dumars, K., J. Burns, S. Kessler, J. Marks, and A. P. Walker. Washington, DC: U. S. Department of Health, Education and Welfare.

Godmilow, L. 1990. "Experience, Intuition are Key." *Perspectives of Genetic Counseling* 12:1.

Gould, S. J. 1985. "Carrie Buck's Daughter." *Constitutional Commentary* 2:331–340.

Greeley, H. T. 1989. "AIDS and the American Health Care Financing System." *University of Pittsburgh Law Review* 51:73–166.

Grice, H. P. 1975. "Logic and Conversation." Pp. 64–78 in *The Logic of Grammar,* edited by Davidson, D. and G. Harman. CA: Wadsworth.

Griswold v. Connecticut 381 U. S. 479 (1965).

Gusella, J., N. S. Wexler, and P. M. Conneally. 1983. "A Polymorphic DNA Marker Genetically Linked to Huntington's Disease." *Nature* 306:234–239.

Haller, M. 1963. *Eugenics: Hereditarian Attitudes in American Thought.* New Brunswick, NJ: Rutgers University Press.

Harding, S. 1986. *The Science Question in Feminism.* Ithaca, NY: Cornell University Press.

Harris, R. 1991. "The New Genetics: A Challenge to Traditional Medicine." *Journal of the Royal College of Physicians of London* 25:134–140.

Heimler, A. 1980. "Opening Remarks: 1980 Business Meeting." *Perspectives in Genetic Counseling* 2:1–2.

Hilts, P. J. 1991. "Groups Set up Panel on Use of Fetal Tissue." *New York Times,* Section B:6(N).

Holmes, S. A. 1991, August 23. "TV Anchor's Disability Stirs Dispute." *The New York Times,* Section A:12.

Holtzman, N. A. 1989. *Proceed with Caution: Predicting Genetic Risks in the Recombinant DNA Era.* Baltimore: Johns Hopkins University Press.

Holtzman, N. A. 1988. "Recombinant DNA Technology, Genetic Tests, and Public Policy." *American Journal of Human Genetics Journal* 42(4):624–632.

Hsia, Y. E. 1979. "The Genetic Counselor as Information Giver." Pp. 169–186 in *Genetic Counseling: Facts, Values and Norms,* edited by Capron, A. M., M. Lappé, R. F. Murrary, T. M. Powledge, S. B. Twiss, and D. Bergsma. New York: Alan R. Liss.

Hubbard, R. 1986. "Eugenics and Prenatal Testing." *International Journal of Health Services* 16:227–242.

Huggins, M., M. Bloch, and S. Kanani. 1990. "Ethical and Legal Dilemmas Arising During Predictive Testing for Adult - Onset Disease: The Experience of Huntington Disease." *American Journal of Human Genetics* 47(1):4–12.

Human Fetal Tissue Transplantation Research Panel. Report Volume I. 1988. Washington DC; *National Institutes of Health.*

Huntington's Disease Society of America. 1989. "Guidelines for Predictive Testing for Huntington's Disease."

Imber, J. 1986. *Abortion and the Private Practice of Medicine.* New Haven: Yale University Press.

International Union United Automobile, Aerospace and Agricultural Implement Workers of America, UAW. 59 LW 4 210. 1991. *Petitioners v. Johnson Controls, Inc.*

International Huntington Association and World Federation of Neurology. 1990. "Ethical Issues Policy Statement on Huntingtons Disease Molecular Genetics Predictive Test." *Journal of Medical Genetics* 27:34–38.

Journal of the House of Representatives, State of Minnesota 1991. 8335.

Kahn, P. L. 1990. "Science and Technology in Public Policy: A Legislator's Perspective Through the Three Branches of Government." *Courts, Health Science & the Law* 1:180–187.

Kamm, F. M. 1986. "Harming, Not Aiding and Positive Rights." *Philosophy of Public Affairs* 15:3–32.

Kearney, W. and A. L. Caplan. 1992. "Parity for Donation." in *Emerging Issues in Biomedical Policy,* edited by Blank, R. and A. Bonnicksen. New York: Columbia University Press.

Kenen, R. 1984. "Genetic Counseling: The Development of a New Interdisciplinary Occupational Field." *Social Science and Medicine* 18:541–549.

Kessler, S., 1980. "The Psychological Paradigm Shift in Genetic Counseling." *Social Biology* 27:167–185.

Kessler, S. and E. K. Levine. 1987. "Psychological Aspects of Genetic Counseling. The Subjective Assessment of Probability." *American Journal of Medical Genetics* 28:361–370.

Kuhn, T. 1977. *The Essential Tension: Selected Studies in Scientific Tradition and Change.* Chicago: University of Chicago Press.

Kushen, R. A. 1988. "Asymptomatic Infection with the AIDS Virus as a Handicap Under the Rehabilitation Act of 1973." *Columbia Law Review* 88:563–586.

LaFave, W. R. and J. H. Israel. 1985. *Criminal Procedure.* St. Paul, MN: West Publishing, Co.

Lehrer, T. 1965. "Wernher von Braun." on That Was the Year That Was, Hollywood: Reprise Records.

Leo, J. 1989. "Genetic Advances, Ethical Risks." *U. S. News & World Report* 59.

Leonard, C. O., G. A. Chase, and B. Childs. 1972. "Genetic Counseling: A Consumer's View." *New England Journal of Medicine* 287:433–439.

Lerman, C., B. Rimer, and F. Engstrom. 1991. "Cancer Risk Notification: Psychological and Ethical Implications." *Journal of Clinical Oncology* 9:127512–127582.

Lewontin, R. C. 1992. "The Dream of the Human Genome." *New York Review of Books* 39:31–40.

Lindemann, E. 1944. "Symptomatology and Management of Acute Grief." *American Journal of Psychiatry* 101:141–148.

Lippman-Hand, A. and F. Clarke Fraser. 1979. "Genetic Counseling–The Post Counseling Period: II. Making Reproductive Choices." *American Journal of Medical Genetics* 4:72–87.

Ludmerer, K. 1972. *Genetics and American Society.* Baltimore: Johns Hopkins University Press.

Markova, I., C. D. Forbes, and M. Inwood. 1979. "The Consumers' View of Genetic Counseling of Hemophilia." *American Journal of Medical Genetics* 17:7417–7452.

Marks, J. H. and M. L. Richter. 1976. "The Genetic Associate: A New Health Professional." *American Journal of Public Health* 66:388–390.

Marks, J. H. and M. L. Richter. 1974. "Training of Genetic Associates." *American Journal of Human Genetics* 26:58A.

McInerney, J. D. 1988. "DNA in Medicine: School-based Education." *Family Journal of Human Genetics* 42:635.

McKusick, V. 1990. *Mendelian Inheritance in Man.* Baltimore: Johns Hopkins University Press.

Menzel, P. 1990. *Strong Medicine: The Ethical Rationing of Health Care.* New Haven: Yale University Press.

Meryash, D. L. and D. Abuelo. 1988. "Counseling Needs and Attitudes Toward Prenatal Diagnosis and Abortion in Fragile-X Families." *Clinical Genetics* 33:349–355.

Mill, J. S. 1874. Pp. 124 in *Essays on Some Unsettled Questions of Political Economy,* edited by Longmans, Green, Reader and Dyer.

Minuchin, S. and H. Fishman. 1981. Pp. 11–27 in *Family Therapy Techniques.* Harvard University Press.

Morris, M. J., A. Tyler, L. Lazarou, L. Meredith, and P. S. Harper. 1989. "Problems in Genetic Prediction for Huntingtons Disease." *The Lancet* 9:601–603.

Müller-Hill, B. 1988. *Murderous Science: Elimination by Scientific Selection of Jews, Gypsies, and Others, Germany 1933–1945.* Oxford: Oxford University Press.

Murray, R. F. 1978. "Genetic Counseling." Pp. 555–566 in *Encyclopedia of Bioethics.* New York: The Free Press.

Murray, R. F. 1974. "The Practitioner's View of the Values Involved in Genetic Screening and Counseling." Pp. 185–199 in *Ethical, Social and Legal Dimensions of Screening for Human Genetic Disease,* edited by J. Bergsma, New York: Stratton.

National Academy of Sciences. 1975. *Genetic Screening: Programs, Principles, and Research.* Washington, DC:

National Center for Human Genome Research. 1990. *The Human Genome Project: New Tools for Tomorrow's Health Research.*

National Society of Genetic Counselors, Inc. (NSGC). 1991b. June. *Code of Ethics*

National Society of Genetic Counselors. 1991a. "Section II: Genetic Counselors and Their Clients." *Code of Ethics*

National Society of Genetic Counselors. 1992. "List of Programs."

National Society of Genetic Counselors. "The Genetic Counselor with a Strong Religious or Spiritual Identity." Workshop presented at Eighth Annual Educational Conference, 1988, New Orleans.

National Commission for the Protection of Human Subjects of Biomedical and Behavioral Research. 1978. September 30. Washington, DC: USGPO.

Nelkin, D. and L. Tancredi. 1989. *Dangerous Diagnostics, The Social Power of Biological Information.* Basic Books.

Neufeld, P. J. and N. Colman. 1990. "When Science Takes the Witness Stand." *Scientific American* 46–53.

Nowak, J. E., R. D. Rotunda, and J. N. Young. 1986. *Constitutional Law.* St. Paul, MN: West Publishing, Co.

Ozawa, C. P. and L. Susskind. 1985. "Mediating Science-Intensive Policy Disputes." *Journal of Policy Analysis and Management* 5:23–39.

Pellegrino, E. and D. Thomasma. 1988. Pp. 141–142 in *For the Patients' Good.* Oxford: Oxford University Press.

Player, M. A. 1988. *Employment Discrimination Law.* St. Paul, MN: West Publishing, Co.

Porter, I. H. 1977. "Evolution of Genetic Counseling in America." in *Genetic Counseling,* edited by Lubs, H. A., and F. dela Cruz. New York: Raven Press.

Powledge, T. 1979. "Genetic Counselors Without Doctorates." Pp. 103–112 in *Genetic Counseling: Facts, Values and Norms,* edited by Capron, A. M., M. Lappé, R. F. Murray. New York: Alan R. Liss.

President's Commission for the Study of Ethical Problems in Medicine and Biomedical and Behavioral Research. 1983a. *Genetic Screening.* Washington: USGPO:

President's Commission for the Study of Ethical Problems in Medicine and Biomedical and Behavioral Research. 1983b. *Screening and Counseling for Genetic Conditions: The Ethical, Social, and Legal Implications of Genetic Screening, Counseling, and Education Programs.* Washington, DC: USGPO.

President's Commission for the Study of Ethical Problems in Medicine and Biomedical and Behavioral Research. 1983c. *Summing Up: The Ethical and Legal Problems in Medicine and Biomedical and Behavioral Research.* Washington, DC: USGPO.

Proctor, R. 1988. *Racial Hygiene: Medicine Under the Nazis.* Cambridge: Harvard University Press.

Quine, W. V. 1960. *Word and Object.* Cambridge: MIT Press.

Rawls, J. 1973. *A Theory of Justice.* Cambridge: Belknap Press of Harvard University Press.

Reed, S. C. 1955. *Counseling in Medical Genetics.* Philadelphia: W. B. Saunders.

Reed, S. C. 1963. *Counseling in Medical Genetics.* Philadelphia: W. B. Saunders, Co.

Reed, S. C. 1980. *Counseling in Medical Genetics.* New York: Alan R. Liss.

Reed, S. C. 1974. "A Short History of Genetic Counseling." *Social Biology* 21:332–339.

Reilly, P. R. 1991. *The Surgical Solution: A History of Involuntary Sterilization in the United States.* Baltimore: Johns Hopkins University Press.

Richter, M. L. 1968. Letter to the Dean of Sarah Lawrence College.

Ritov, I. and J. Baron. 1990. "Reluctance to Vaccinate: Omission Bias and Ambiguity." *Journal of Behavioral Decision Making* 3:263–277.

Roberts, L. 1990. "To Test or Not to Test?" *Science* 247:17–19.

Rogers, C. R. 1951. *Client-Centered Therapy: Its Current Practice, Implications, and Theory.* Boston: Houghton Mifflin.

Rollnick, B. R. 1984. "The NSGC: An Historical Perspective." Pp. 3–7 in *Strategies in Genetic Counseling: Clinical Investigation Studies,* edited by Fine, B. A., and N. W. Paul. New York: March of Dimes Birth Defects Foundation.

Root, M. 1992. *The Liberal Sciences: Seeking the Facts and Hiding the Values.* (Chapter 9). Work in Progress, .

Rothman, B. K. 1986. *The Tentative Pregnancy: Prenatal Diagnosis and the Future of Motherhood.* New York: Penguin Books.

Rucher, R. and A. Strauss. 1961. "Professions in Process." *American Journal of Sociology* 66:325–334.

Schatz, B. 1987. "The AIDS Insurance Crisis: Underwriting or Overreaching." *Harvard Law Review* 100:1782–1805.

Sellars, M. 1982. "Ethical Aspects of Genetic Counseling." *Journal of Medical Ethics* 8:185–188.

Sherry, S. 1984. "Selective Judicial Activism in the Equal Protection Context: Democracy, Distrust, and Deconstruction." *Georgetown Law Journal* 73:89–125.

Shoop, T. 1991. "Biology's Moon Shot." *Government Executive* 10–17.

Skoglund, W. J. 1991. Letter to Phyllis L. Kahn.

Sly, W. S. 1973. "What is Genetic Counseling?" In *Contemporary Genetic Counseling,* edited by Bergsma, D. White Plains, NY: The National Foundation-March of Dimes.

Solnit, J. A. and M. H. Stark. 1961. "Mourning and the Birth of a Defective Child." *Psychoanalytic Study of the Child* 16:523–527.

Sorenson, J. R., J. Swazey, and N. Scotch. 1981. Pp. 132–41 *Reproductive Past Reproductive Futures.* March of Dimes.

Sorenson, J. R. 1976. "From Social Movement to Clinical Medicine: The Role of Law and the Medical Profession in Regulating Applied Human Genetics." Pp. 474 in *Genetics and the Law.* New York: Plenum Press.

Sorenson, J. R. and A. Culbert. 1977. "Genetic Counselors and Counseling Orientations-Unexamined Topics in Evaluation." Pp. 131–56 in *Genetic Counseling,* edited by Lubs, H. A. and F. de la Cruz. New York: Raven Press.

Sorenson, J. R., C. M. Kavanagh, and M. Mucatel. 1981. "Client Learning of Risk and Diagnosis in Genetic Counseling." in *The Fetus and the Newborn,* edited by Bloom, A. D., L. S. James, and N. W. Paul. New York: Alan R. Liss.

Specter, M. 1990. "Abortion Issue Chills Research: Fetal Tissue Ban Sidelines US Experts." *Washington Post,* Section A:8.

State v. Kim 398 N. W. 2d 544 (1987).

State v Schwartz 447, N. W. 2d 422 (1989).

Tauer, C. 1990. "Human Fetal Tissue: Scientific Uses and Ethical Concerns." *Journal of the Minnesota Academy of Science* 55:2–9.

Thompson, J. S. and M. W. Thompson, Ed. 1986. Pp. 1–3 in *Genetics in Medicine,* Philadelphia: W. B. Saunders.

Tribe, L. H. 1988. *American Constitutional Law.* Mineola, NY: The Foundation Press.

Twiss, S. B. 1979. "The Genetic Counselor as Moral Advisor." Pp. 201–212 in *Genetic Counseling: Fact, Values and Norms,* edited by Capron, A. M., M. Lappé, R. F. Murray. New York: Alan R. Liss.

U. S. Congress Office of Technology Assessment. 1988. *Mapping Our Genes.* Washington, DC: USGPO.

United States President's Commission for the Study of Ethical Problems in Medicine and Biomedical and Behavioral Research. 1982.

Walker, A. P., J. A. Scott, B. B. Biesecker, B. Conover, W. Blake, and L. Djurdjinovic. 1990. "Report of the 1989 Asilomar Meeting on Education in Genetic Counseling." *American Journal of Human Genetics* 46:1223–1230.

Warren, K. J. 1987. "Feminism and Ecology: Making Connections." *Environmental Ethics* 9:3–20.

Wertz, D. C. and J. C. Fletcher. 1988a. "Attitudes of Genetic Counselors: A Multi-National Survey." *American Journal of Human Genetics* 42:592–600.

Wertz, D. C. and J. C. Fletcher. 1988b. "Ethics and Medical Genetics in the United States: A National Survey." *American Journal of Human Genetics* 29:815–827.

Wertz, D. C. and J. C. Fletcher. 1989. *Ethics and Human Genetics: A Cross-Cultural Perspective*. Berlin and New York: Springer-Verlag.

Wertz, D. C., C. Fletcher, and J. J. Mulvihill. 1990. "Medical Geneticists Confront Ethical Dilemmas: Cross Cultural Comparisons Among 18 Nations." *American Journal of Human Genetics* 46:1200–1213.

Wertz, D. C., J. M. Rosenfield, and S. R. Janes. 1991. "Attitudes Toward Abortion Among Parents of Children with Cystic Fibrosis." *American Journal of Public Health* 81:992–996.

West, R. 1988. "Ethical Aspects of Genetic Disease and Genetic Counseling." *Journal of Medical Ethics* 14:194–197.

World Medical Association. 1987. "Statement on Genetic Counseling and Genetic Engineering." *IME Bulletin* 31:8–9.

Wright, E. E. 1978. "Father and Mother Know Best: Defining the Liability of Physicians for Inadequate Genetic Counseling." *Yale Law Journal* 87:1488–1515.

Yarborough, M., J. Scott, and L. Dixon. 1989. "The Role of Beneficence in Clinical Genetics: Nondirective Counseling Reconsidered." *Theoretical Medicine* 10:139–148.

Index